Toxic Overload

Why Are We a Sick Society?

A Breakthrough Program to Prevent & Reverse the Causes of Disease at Any Age

Dr. Harold Steinberg

Table of Contents

Dedication

The future is in the hands of our children and their children. A good and peaceful world is in their hands. So, I want to dedicate this book to all children, in all countries, of all nationalities who are affected by the toxic onslaughts of the chemical invasion of their bodies. They are the future of our planet and need to be made aware of what is affecting their health.

Children Learn What They Live
By Dorothy Law Nolte, Ph.D.

If children live with criticism, they learn to condemn.
If children live with hostility, they learn to fight.
If children live with fear, they learn to be apprehensive.
If children live with pity, they learn to feel sorry for themselves.
If children live with ridicule, they learn to feel shy.
If children live with jealousy, they learn to feel envy.
If children live with shame, they learn to feel guilty.
If children live with encouragement, they learn confidence.
If children live with tolerance, they learn patience.
If children live with praise, they learn appreciation.
If children live with acceptance, they learn to love.
If children live with approval, they learn to like themselves.
If children live with recognition, they learn it is good to have a goal.
If children live with sharing, they learn generosity.
If children live with honesty, they learn truthfulness.
If children live with fairness, they learn justice.
If children live with kindness and consideration, they learn respect.
If children live with security, they learn to have faith in themselves
and in those about them.
If children live with friendliness, they learn the world is a nice place
in which to live.

1

Mission

The mission of the St. Francis Chiropractic Health Clinic is to find the cause of the patient's illness, pain and discomfort. With the input of their laboratory blood and urine reports, X-rays, MRI, and the Bio-Detoxification questionnaire, if needed, plus the biofeedback reports showing the specific sensitivities from the bio-system analysis, we can look at the biochemical and structural causes of their problems.

We are treating the patient and not the disease. We look at the constitution of the patient, how long have they been sick, and how encumbered are they with toxins and/or pathogens.

Once the source of the problem is determined, we can customize the use of homeopathy, herbs, supplements and real food to correct and stabilize the problems.

We may incorporate chiropractic adjustments, acupuncture meridian recommendations, dental hygiene, emotional techniques and exercise programs to achieve the goal of restoring the vitality to the patient's nervous system; and gently support the elimination of toxins and pathogens as an effective way to downregulate inflammation and modulate the immune system.

The care the patients receive is tailored to their needs. The patient is the individual we are working with. Each patient is different from other individuals and is treated as such. The holistic approaches to the patient's health needs are the nervous, immune and endocrine systems plus diet, lifestyle and emotional needs. If the patient is interested in improving their health, we will provide the means and information to do so in a one on one environment. The conversation of disease starts with the statement that disease is caused by inflammation and stress. These can be eliminated with knowledge and a change in lifestyle. We are serious about helping the patient achieve optimal health and wellness.

Introduction

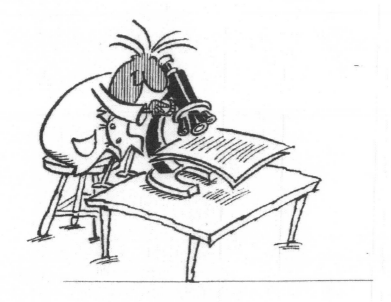

Everyone is different, each a mystery to solve.

For all the years in practice I have spoken to my patients about nutrition, chiropractic and how the body heals. When there have been health questions I reviewed their blood lab work and made nutritional suggestions where appropriate.

With all the nutritional help and prescription aids I have not seen major improvements in their health. Their health is declining. Looking at the reports of the health of people in the US we are not healthier. Looking at longevity charts, the people in the US are not living long in relation to the rest of the world. So, the question to ask is why is this happening?

Not all patients get well when put on a prescription drug routine or on a nutritional program. This led me to start to think out of the box.

What are the important factors to look at in determining the success of a nutritional wellness practice to help people rid themselves of chronic diseases, stay healthy and achieve longevity?

The first factor is understanding that all patients have unique biochemical individuality and the second factor is they all have been, and still are, exposed to a large number of toxins in their daily lives.

Can toxins affect a person's health, mentally and/or physically? The answer is an absolute yes.

We will review where these toxins are, what they are and make suggestions on how to limit their usage, list the sources of the problem and how to rid them from our bodies. We will be referring to a bio communications program which is an instrumental tool in the work we do.

We are lucky to be in a country where food is plentiful; where we are not lacking drinking water, where there are thousands of pharmacies, where there are thousands of vitamin and natural health stores; where there are hundreds of thousands of prescriptions and over the counter drugs and hundreds of thousands of supplements for every ailment; where the medical treatments and hospitals are exceptional.

This is a country where food producers will put unhealthy and even unsafe chemicals in their food products to reduce the cost, increase the products shelf life and increase profits.

Try an experiment with a piece of bread or a few grains or flakes of cold cereal. Place it on the ground outside your house and see how many minutes, hours, days or weeks it will still be there.

The last time I did the test, I had to pick up the test "food" and throw it away after two weeks. No animal or insect would eat the piece of bread or cereal flakes.

This is a country where the pharmaceutical companies inundate us with drugs, vaccinations, and products that will cure almost anything. They are advertised on the TV by the dozens. As we all know the drugs do cost a lot of money in this country and many people can't afford them.

So, with all of this great food and pharmaceuticals I need to ask the question, WHY ARE WE STILL A SICK SOCIETY? WHAT ARE WE MISSING?

After many years of research and working with my patients I believe the answer to why we are a sick society will be covered in this book. Discussions of digestion are important as well as the nature of detox, to how we can stay healthy. The method of food creation, the use of pesticides, the chemicals in our drinking and bathing water, the failing regulatory role of the EPA to control toxic chemical waste products in the air, water, land and foods, the toxic chemicals in our body lotions and crèmes and potions, the chemicals in our clothing and furniture plus the genetically modified foods will add much to the answer of why we are sick.

Chapter 1 - Society is Killing Us

"Great spirits have always encountered violent opposition from mediocre minds"

Albert Einstein

In my research, experience in my nutritional practice, reading scientific journals and attending seminars I became aware of the fact that society is killing us.

This does sound preposterous, but it is true. What we are doing in our daily life is having a detrimental effect on our health. We are bombarded with chemicals, pesticides, preservatives, foods, prescriptions and over the counter drugs never before imaginable. These are powerful chemical insults imposed on our bodies every minute of every day. These insults are toxins that are harmful agents found in the environment and are accumulating in our human body, and in our animal friends, causing disease, ill health and stress and inflammation.

Blood tests done at the Center for Disease Control have found hundreds of these toxic chemicals in our blood. The items found are acrylamide, from foods that are baked or fried at high temperatures, BPA, arsenic and herbicides, pesticides, insecticides, personal care products and dry-cleaning materials. These are but a few of the daily toxins.

What about bacteria, viruses, parasites and molds? A point not to be missed are the large amounts of vaccinations, over the counter drugs and pharmaceutical drugs people are taking. The opioid epidemic is growing out of hand.

The scary part of these drugs are the numbers each person is taking. It is now called poly-pharmacology. We know, maybe the working pathway of a drug, but what about two, three or ten drugs that people are taking? The earliest involvement I had with this concept was reading Rachel Carson's "Silent Spring". My reading of the book was many decades ago, but I had not forgotten her message. She wrote about the negative effects of poisons in our environment. Maybe that was the start of the Environmental Protection Agency?

9

Since that time many more authors have written articles and books about the impact on society and people from chemicals in our foods and clothing and the environment.

The control of many environmental toxins was implemented under the Obama administration and now under the present administration in 2017, the EPA department is reversing the controls on the toxins and chemicals that can or are affecting the health and wellness of millions of people in the US and the rest of the world.

The Trump/Pence/Pruitt administration is disallowing scientific study in favor of monetary gain for corporations. All the work done earlier is being cancelled, or is to be cancelled, and industry is allowed to operate freely. The caring for the people's health is being withdrawn for the sake of profit.

What the chemical companies are blind to is the effect these poisons have on everybody in the USA, the adjacent countries and even the world. Air, water and food wind up in other countries and can have negative effects on all people. The toxins they create have an effect on all of us. The chemical poisons that are created in the name of advancement of science, and profit, don't know the difference between the poor and wealthy. How long will these poisons stay active in the soil or in the air or in the waters?

Dangerous Chemicals in the Environment:

The growth of diseases, specifically auto immune and cancer, should be a concern for everybody. We all don't have to be scientists to understand that chemicals can disrupt our life by affecting our hormonal (endocrine) systems. Many of these chemicals are listed on the labels of the foods we eat, the lotions put on our bodies and the cleaning products we use daily. The chemicals do have long and complicated names, but we need to be aware of them. There is no reason to hide from chemicals that can affect our health and our lives.

There are hundreds, if not thousands, of chemicals that can affect our endocrine systems which can affect our reproductive capability, migraine headaches, weight gain, and our "feeling good" in general. A summary of 13 toxic substances are listed below. This should keep you reading about other potent chemicals in our environment.

1.   Phthalates are hormone disruptors and are xenoestrogenic, meaning they are synthetic mimickers of estrogen, which contributes to cancer of the breast. They are found in some soft plastic water bottles, nail polish and lacquers.

2.   Propylene Glycol is antifreeze. It is used in body lotions and cosmetics.

3.   Parabens or Methylparaben is also xenoestrogenic and can contribute to cancer of the breast. Try to buy paraben free products.

4.   Sodium Laurel Sulfate is found in toothpaste, shampoos and cleansers. Read the labels of all the products, even natural products can have SLS in it.

5.   Bisphenol A, BPA, has xenoestrogenic effects on men and women reproductive systems. BPA is in plastics and is used as linings in canned soups, beans and vegetables. Replace with glass packed or ceramic lined cans. Again, you need to read labels.

6.   Bisphenol S, BPS have health issues as BPA. Thermal receipt paper is the culprit.

7.   Triclosan can increase androgens, the male sex hormone and reduce or depress estrogen. Triclosan is found in hand sanitizers and in anti-bacterial soaps.

8.   Formaldehyde can be carcinogenic, can affect menstrual cycles, and can irritate eyes and skin. It can be found in air fresheners, hair sprays and nail polish.

9.   Chlorine can be connected to low thyroid functions, endometriosis, endocrine disorders, and low sperm count. Chlorine is found in dish detergents and in public water supplies. In swimming pools and in drinking water from the tap and in bottled water.

10.   Sodium Hydroxide which can irritate eyes, damage skin and irritate lungs and throat. It is found in oven cleaners.

11.   Perchloroethylene is a VOC, volatile organic compound, that can affect lungs and cause respiratory illness. It can have long term kidney and fetus effects. VOC's are found in carpet cleaners, shoe polish, dry cleaning chemicals, paint removers and adhesives.

12.   Fragrance like perfume is another xenoestrogenic problem. This is found in cosmetics, hair products, household cleaners, air fresheners, scented menstrual pads, and scented trash bags. The word fragrance on a label can really contain many different chemicals.

13.   Fluoride and Bromine are also connected to low thyroid function. These chemicals are used in swimming pools, in public drinking water and in most bottle waters. Fluoride in toothpastes and mouth washes do not reduce dental cavities many studies have shown.

Early Ancestors:

Our ancestors did not live in the world we are now living in. Centuries ago there were no man made chemical toxins to affect their bodies. There were poisonous plants, snakes, other animals, sea life and mushrooms. The plants and fruits made their own protective chemicals to keep themselves from being attacked by insects or animals.

Now we are generating the pesticides and chemicals through "better living through chemistry". The question we need to ponder is, are we able to cope with all the insults affecting our body daily?

Chemicals, like pesticides, vaccinations with heavy metals and preservatives, Rx drugs and OTC drugs are bombarding our bodies with toxins we are not aware of, are not tested for, and we don't know how to detox from.

Our illnesses become a vicious cycle and every day we add to the level of chemical toxicity the body needs to cope with. These toxins are in our water, our food, our homes, our clothes and in the air we breathe. It is a cycle we need to be aware of.

Ingested Toxins:

Drugs of any kind and even the best supplements, herbs and homeopathic products can return us to apparent good health, but we need to put an effort toward putting clean foods into our bodies and removing the toxins we are ingesting.

We need to get companies to remove all the toxic additives they use in "living better through chemistry". These chemical toxins lead to poor health, inflammation, stress and anxiety and that leads to disease and death. The toxins are affecting the nutrition from our foods, imposing larger demands on our immune system, and stressing our detox functions in our livers and affecting the normal function of our digestion.

It is difficult to be as healthy as our ancestors when our body is fighting chemicals and toxins that have been newly introduced to our system.

Years ago, I looked at the pieces that made up diseases. Since a lot of these involved transmission through the blood and lymph system I gave it the name "the hot house" principle. The premise was clear that the body's fight was on against those invaders. The pH was altered, and the body needed to balance the pH of the blood and tissues to fight a winning battle. The steps involved in creating disease is shown in the chart below.

HOT HOUSE EFFECT

IF PH
UNBALANCED:

THINGS 'GROW':

MOLD   FUNGUS

VIRUSES

BACTERIA

PARASITES   CANDIDA

DISEASE BLOSSOMS AND GROWS

A BALANCED CHEMISTRY IS A HAPPY BODY

Add to this chart **Environmental Toxins, Water Contaminates, Food Preservatives, Air Pollution, Vaccinations, Antibiotics, and Body/Cosmetic toxins** and we are affecting our health as we have not in the past. These add up to be stressful to the body and lead to inflammation, which over time leads to disease conditions. Other notable areas of stress are our life style, work, home issues, news, war, salary and housing are contributors to stress which can lead to disease states. Other causes of disease are society's rules and regulations for the way we manufacture and process food products, household products used for cleaning, body cleaning items and chemicals.

The question we need to ask is can our body handle these strange toxic insults with our inherent immune system? If the answer is no, then the question is how can we remove these toxins from our bodies? Is there a protocol out there that will assist us? I found a tool that can assist us in the process of toxin removal and help our body get a handle on these poisons and assist the body in eliminating them from our system and minimize their life-threatening toxins. It is necessary to evaluate everyone as an individual. The personalized approach is designed for you, your personal life style and your personalized protocols. We will expand on these during the book.

Questions of Detox:

Can we develop the mechanisms to detox, dissolve and eliminate these chemicals before they cause major harm to us, our children, their children and society as a whole?

This is more than a simple issue. We are gambling with chemistry and gene modification that can have devastating effects on the health and wellbeing of the society we know. What if it takes more than a decade to see epigenetic changes? What if it takes a generation to make epigenetic changes?

We are learning a lot about genetics and the role it may play in diseases. But can we change the genetics with mass influxes of chemicals and pesticides? Are we playing a game of roulette at speeds we can't imagine? I am not just talking about this year. What happens when a couple marries and has children? What is the combined effect on the siblings? What about the next generation and the next? Are we creating a problem with no solution?

Epigenetics:

Epigenetics is the environmental impact on our genetics. The definition of epigenetics is: *relating to, being, or involving changes in gene function that do not involve changes in DNA sequence.*

Will things in the environment affect our genes negatively? Genes can be "activated" by the impact of toxins in our environment. When insults from chemicals are imposed on our genes what happens? Do the genes change and make us sick, weak, or become diseased?

Studies have been done by scientists to show that the chemicals in our environment, in our workplace, in our homes, in our daily cleaning products and beauty products can change our genes and affect our long-term health.

Will the chemicals in the environment activate the "bad" dormant genes and cause disease conditions to awaken? Yes, is the answer. Many scientists think these toxins can cause a decrease in the state of health of humans and animals we have not experienced in decades.

What about the millions and millions of bacteria in all of us? They play an integral part in our health and nutrition. They are affected by the toxins and if they are modified or reduced in number they will also affect our health status to the negative.

Another issue to ponder is that scientists are also concerned about the earth's warming state. Will melting ice and defrosting of the tundra release bacteria and viruses that we have not been exposed to for millennia?

The Future - Offspring:

With the union of couples creating offspring with these genetic insults, what have they created? Maybe disease states we have never seen before. More autistic kids. More cancer. More autoimmune diseases. These cases and numbers will be tracked by health workers around the world.

Can these toxins put stress on gene encoding that in turn can lead to disease states? Can these toxins affect our mitochondria and create vulnerability to degenerative diseases like Alzheimer's? Can they cause genetic mutations? Some genes will adapt to stress from all these known pressures and environmental changes that are new to our genomes.

The CDC Analysis:

The CDC did find these toxins do accumulate in our blood and in our tissues. How can we rid the body of these chemical burdens? The organs we need to employ are our liver and kidneys. But they can be overwhelmed with the magnitude of the job to break down and eliminate chemicals toxins that are man-made. We need to add the immune system to this elimination pathway to assist the body to build resources against these toxins.

Chapter 2 - How Digestion Works

"Bad digestion is the root of all evil" – Hippocrates

The process of digestion is so much a normal daily function we normally do not think of the steps involved in the digestion process.

First there is chewing of foods we are eating. The teeth are designed for chewing. The anterior, or front, teeth are to provide the cutting action and the molars, or back, teeth provide the grinding action. The foods must be broken down.

Chewing of the food is important for digestion of all foods. The membranes around cells must be broken down before the food nutrition can be utilized. Chewing aids in the digestion of food for the following simple reason because the digestive enzymes act only on the surface of food particles. The rate of digestion is highly dependent on the total surface area exposed to the internal secretions of enzymes and acids. The more food is chewed the easier the food moves from the stomach into the small intestine and the rest of the gut.

As a practitioner of functional medicine, the gut is at the center of most all disease conditions. The gut is referred to as the second brain. Digestive stress can lead to a condition called leaky gut or intestinal permeability which can lead to autoimmune disease and other diseases.

When we normally think of autoimmunity we think of the body attacking itself. For example, Hashimoto's is the body attacking the thyroid gland. What causes this to happen? Can autoimmunity be part of the body nutrient depletion that occurs with poor digestion or by drug induced nutrient depletion. Nutrient depletion is covered in Chapter 4.

In the study of biochemistry, we learned that there are specific nutritional elements needed for a healthy thyroid, adrenals, kidney and liver to perform at peak efficiency. We learned that hundreds of enzyme reactions in our cells need specific nutrients and illnesses may occur when the nutrition is not provided.

Most people need to revisit the anatomy of their bodies to recall how we digest foods and the organs involved in that process. The following diagram is a review of the digestive system.

The importance of that system is that is how we process all the food we consume, all the water we drink, all the chemicals that are in the foods we eat, all the vitamins and supplements we take, and all the pharmaceutical and over the counter drugs we consume.

The chemicals and toxins and even the food particles, after digestion, can enter the blood system through a procedure called leaky gut, where food particles are now using the effort of our immune system to fight the food and not the real enemies of bacteria, viruses, mold, parasites and diseases.

Once these toxins are in the blood they can affect all organs and even the brain. So, a good question to ask is how is your gut? And what do you eat or drink? A reason for this question is that all foods and chemicals need to be processed, in a detox mode, by the liver. The more toxins processed the more burden and stress is imposed on the liver.

The gut, or stomach and small intestines, are the second brain. Most of the neurotransmitters the brain needs are created in the gut. Proteins are broken down into amino acids which become the neurotransmitters the brain needs. Serotonin and melatonin are two important products needed to help sleep and mental stability. When the biological processing system is modified we get strange physiological results. For example, when stomach acid is limited or totally eliminated, it is difficult for the body to break down protein food sources and then the production of neurotransmitters is limited, and people can experience mental health deficiencies. Stress, depression and suicidal tendencies may be the result. The book, "The Mood Cure" by Julia Ross covers amino acid needs by the body to balance emotional issues.

The first diagram shows the organs that make up the digestive system. The second diagram shows the levels of acidity needed for the body to function properly. Each part needs to contribute for the engine to run properly. The removal of an organ surgically, like the gall bladder, has an effect on digestion. This can be compensated for with the right knowledge of supplements and/or diet changes.

Anatomy of a Digestive System

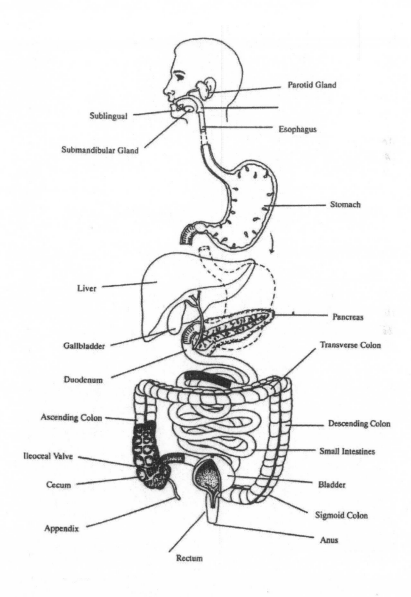

How The Digestive System Works

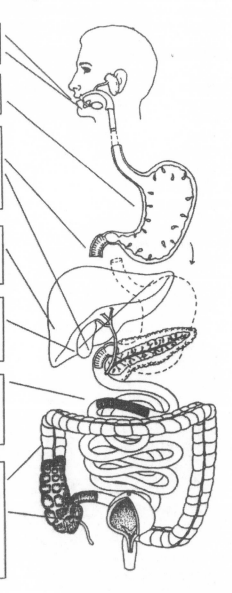

Food enters the mouth. Salivary glands secrete alkaline saliva (8.0 ph) containing enzymes to mix with food.

Hydrochloric acid (0.8 pH) created by parietal cells activates pepsinogen enzymes and mixes with food.

Food passes through the pyloric valve and moves past the highly alkaline Brunners glands (8.9 pH) and into duodenum. Here the alkaline pancreatic juices (8.3 pH), full of enzymes, enter the duodenum along with alkaline gall juices (bile)(8.6 pH). With a healthy person, the food mixture (chyme) now becomes alkaline.

Liver provides alkalinity for saliva and creates bile. All food that is assimilated will go through the liver and the liver will detoxify harmful substances and produce the final preparations for use throughout the body.

·Bile is stored in the gall bladder. If necessary the body will extract organic sodium from the bile and use it in other areas. The bile pH will drop when this occurs and gallstones may be formed.

Small intestines produce even more alkalinity from the crypts of Lieberkuhn and more than 22 other enzymes gradually mix with the food, if the guts are clear of mucoid plaque. Then the small intestines gradually assimilate digested food.

Food moves out of the small intestines through the ileocecal valve and into the cecum. This is a sight where many parasites dwell in unhealthy people. Then the food moves up through the ascending colon, through the transverse colon and down the descending colon, past the sigmoid, rectum, and out the anus. The sigmoid and rectum are among the most common sites of cancer and other bowel diseases in constipated individuals.

Stomach Acid:

Stomach acid is the body's first line of defense to protect itself from food or drink that carry bacteria, viruses or molds

With all the acid inhibitors sold as prescriptions or as OTC products we have lost this first line of defense. The concept of all the people taking antacids having too much stomach acid says that we were not created with a good design and there are thousands of people that are creating too much stomach acid.

Could the problem be the crappy foods we are eating? Could it be the drugs we are taking? Could it be the result of the small intestine bacteria releasing enzymes to digest the undigested food in our stomach or small intestine? Could it be too much liquids ingested with our meals which dilute the stomach acid and result in less digestion? Could it be we are not chewing enough to reduce the foods to small pieces to be easily digested? It could be any, or all, of the above elements that create the heartburn that causes discomfort.

Whether it is processed foods, genetically modified organisms (GMO) foods, preservatives added to foods or the way foods are prepared, these may be the reasons why we can't digest foods the way our bodies were designed to do.

It is easier to write a prescription for an acid inhibitor than to explain issues that can affect the patients' health in the short term, and more importantly in the long term. As doctors, we need to teach patients how to stay healthy. The concept of how we digest food is what we all learn in school. To modify the steps in the digestive process without explaining it to the patient makes no sense.

It is like removing the gallbladder with no explanation of what the gallbladder does and what the patient needs to do after the removal of the gallbladder. Stomach acid is needed to digest protein, create amino acids and breakdown minerals to be an absorbable element. The protein breakdown to amino acids is necessary to create neurotransmitters in the intestines that are then transmitted to the brain. The minerals are needed as catalysts or cofactors for the thousands of enzymatic reactions that occur in all cells.

When we stop the body's natural creation of stomach acid, we are creating muscle wasting, malnutrition due to a lack of protein breakdown, mineral deficiencies and even neurological disorders like anxiety, depression and even suicidal tendencies. Can dementia and Alzheimer's disease be a result of a lack of stomach acid?

The acid reducing prescriptions and over the counter products suppress our own acid production. Stomach acid is needed to break down foods, especially proteins we eat. The normal reaction of the health care community is to write a script for an acid reducer when a patient complains about acid reflux. The problem is not too much acid, it is too little acid.

Because of low B12 the body can't produce enough stomach acid. Without stomach acid the body can't extract iron from food and B12 from food thus creating digestive problems and health problems since we need iron for carrying oxygen in our red blood cells and we need B12 for acid production and neurological balance. As you can see in the following chart there are many other vitamins and minerals that are not processed without stomach acid.

For example, Vitamin K is for blood clotting. Zinc is for our immune system.

Good intestinal Flora	Selenium
Boron	Thiamin
Chromium	Vitamin B12
Copper	Vitamin C
Digestive acids Folic acid	Vitamins D & E
Iron	Vitamins K
Phosphorous	Zinc

The removal of the gallbladder and the elimination of stomach acid can affect the nature of what foods are being digested. The small and large   intestines are packed with intestinal bacteria which are responsible for extracting vitamins from our foods. The type of food we eat can change the bacterial makeup in our intestines. High carbohydrate foods, and different prescription medicines, like birth control oral contraceptives, antibiotics and acid suppressing drugs affect the type and balance of the intestinal bacteria.

Liver's Role in Detox:

A conversation with patients about nutrition is an important part of their education. We do discuss digestion and how it works. We do ask about the prescription drugs they are taking. This is covered in the section on "Drug Induced Nutrient Depletion". We also speak about the importance of the liver and its detox functions. The liver is one of the body's most essential organs. It filters blood and metabolizes nutrients and detoxes chemicals and drugs. Most patients know the word "detox". An explanation of detox is important as well as the understanding of the two steps, or phases, in the detox process. A list of the vitamins and minerals needed for detox and nutrition for the phase are listed below.

Phase 1: this phase metabolizes pharmaceutical and recreational drugs by creating free radicals. There is a family of enzymes called cytochrome P450 that performs phase 1 transformations. The P450 makes toxins water soluble and converts toxins into less toxic molecules.

B vitamins – from whole food sources

Vitamins A, C, and E

Flavonoids from fruits and vegetables

Glutathione

Alpha-lipoic acid

Milk Thistle or Silymarin

Vitamin E and Selenium

Phospholipids in eggs, meat, soybean, fish

Phase 2: this phase protects against chemical carcinogens. It initiates heavy metal detoxification and recycles CoQ10, which is a potent antioxidant.

Glutathione

Fish oil – omega 3

Amino acids – all the essentials ones the body can't make

Probiotics and fiber

Cabbage and broccoli and cruciferous vegetables

Limonene in lemons, dill and oranges

Supplements for Us and Pets:

In addition to good foods you may need to add high quality "food based supplements" made from real foods and not from petrochemical sources. When you think of petrochemicals, think of using petroleum to make a chemical representation of the vitamin which are then ingested.

Reduce your toxic load by changing your eating habits and purchase products that are safer with less chemical toxins. Read labels and be conscious of what products you put on your body and what you put in your body. Be especially conscious of what you use on your kid's bodies and what you put in their bodies. This can also be applied to your pets. As far as foods are concerned, more carbohydrates and less protein may not be a healthy mix for your loved pets. Be aware of the foods you are feeding them and the products you spray or put on their bodies.

It is important to rid your body of these toxins before they cause illness and diseases. The importance of good and clean foods and supplements is to feed the liver and kidneys with the nutrition they need to stay healthy and be ahead of the game. Their performance matters in our cleansing and health.

Chapter 3 – Disease State & Cause of Disease

Disease condition:

Many years ago, I became interested in finding a way to determine if a disease condition can be found many years prior to the disease appearing later in life. My goal is not to diagnose the name of the disease, but what are the causes of the disease.

The body, your body, knows how healthy it is and what it needs to stay healthy. What we need is a tool or system to communicate with the body/brain and listen to what it is saying. There is a mechanism available, called biofeedback, or bio communication, which addresses the communication to your body and helps achieve health. It is based on quantum frequency energy and may be a step in our health future of medicine. We will explain and show examples later in the book.

Cause of Disease:

What is the cause of disease? Is it one condition or is it a combination of steps that accumulate and result in a disease condition? Many scientists and medical professionals have written papers on the causes of disease. The latest thoughts are that diseases are a result of stress and inflammation. But what is the cause of that stress and inflammation? Do we know what is the factor or factors that influence stress or inflammation to occur?

These conditions can be from physical or emotional causes that are recent or can go back to when we were children. Could the cause of disease include bacteria, viruses, mold, fungus or parasites?

Many scientists feel these, together with environmental chemicals, drugs and pesticides are a major contributor of inflammation and disease.

Degenerative Diseases:

Burton Goldberg in Alternative Medicine, November 1999, wrote that "It usually takes years, often decades, of development, before degenerative diseases manifest themselves.

Using alternative medical diagnosis techniques, you can identify trouble brewing far in advance, and take steps to avoid disease altogether." His article described three areas of importance. He specified darkfield microscopy, electrodermal screening (EDS) and thermography.

As part of my practice I added the darkfield and EDS with nutritional consulting to learn about interpreting blood and urine tests. I recently added the latest EDS computerized system, called decision support, to the practice.

Initially I followed the suggested uses of nutritional protocols. Some of the patients were helped for a short period of time and then the old symptoms reappeared. I thought the problem we were trying to solve was a symptom that may be a result of another and deeper problem. More lab tests were done by their physicians. The same "you are normal" was the usual result. "It's in your head". Blood and urine tests have ranges of numbers that cover the 95% normal and 5% ill in a very large population. Most are told by their physicians they are in the normal range, but they still are not feeling well.

When we test blood in the laboratory we get a reading of the markers that are in the blood now. The ranges of the markers get wider, or in some cases get narrower, to emphasize some medical hypothesis.

The tests used by laboratory analysis of blood does show CRP (C - reactive protein) for inflammation condition or an infection and ESR (Erythrocyte Sedimentation Rate).

With urine, the analysis is the family of white blood cells that show increases in active viral or bacterial infection when the total WBC number increases. Monocytes will show increases in inflammation or parasites. Eosinophils, when increased, can indicate parasites or allergy sensitivities. The increase of basophils indicates inflammatory or parasitic conditions. Increased neutrophils and lymphocytes can mean active infections.

But where is the stress? What organ system is it addressing? The biofeedback system can evaluate the stresses in one's body and will use supplements, foods, minerals, vitamins and homeopathy to rid the body of stress, anxiety and inflammation before it leads to a diseased state.

It is not the Tricorder of Star Trek but it is pretty close. The biofeedback system uses a functional medicine approach instead of a symptom medical approach.

Are Lab Tests the Truth?

Looking at blood and urine lab work doesn't always answer why you are feeling poorly. "When medical tests mislead" is an article in the December 2016 issue of Scientific American. The author, Charles Schmidt, discusses the fact that the FDA is cracking down on medically questionable lab tests (blood).

"We tend to think of lab tests as being the ultimate truth," says Ramy Arnaout of Harvard Medical School. "But no test is 100 percent accurate, and some of the LDTs (lab-developed tests) aren't medically useful at all."

The closing paragraph should open our thought process. It states "For patients and their physicians, the question is much more basic. Why should we ever have to wonder whether a commercially available medical test does more harm than good?"

Another point about lab test ranges is, are they representative of a patient's health? The ranges from low to high vary based upon many factors. The one that has varied the most is total cholesterol level. Originally it was 180 – 260. Sometimes the upper end range was stated as 100 plus the patient's age. Then it was reduced to upper range of 240. Then to 220. The most recent printed range for cholesterol is 100-199.

We need cholesterol for brain function and for nerve insulation. The Mayo Clinic does not want levels so low. It can have detrimental effects on memory, heart health and can lead to cancer and this low end is considered in the normal range.

Nutrition and Detox:

Discussions about diet and nutrition do not normally occur in the medical office. The topic of detox doesn't get covered. Prescription drugs are offered as a solution that does not always address the health condition. When you think about pain pills or over the counter drugs have you thought about why not use more natural products to resolve pain? What about disease states? Can we use foods, vitamins and minerals and herbs to attack or limit disease, pain or stress and inflammatory conditions? The answer is a resounding yes.

Chapter 4 - Drug Induced Nutrient Depletion

Our healing concept is to provide nutritional supplementation through foods, vitamins and minerals, herbs and homeopathy to improve your health before using OTC or Rx drugs.

The nutritional approach is extremely important for people taking pharmaceutical drugs. There is a very important reason to impress people to add nutrition to their diets. Drugs tend to eliminate nutrients from the body. I never tell people to get off prescription drugs. But knowing the body can't improve without replenishing the nutrients, I look at reinforcing the body with nutrients the drugs remove from the body. Otherwise, the health of the individual is in a health decline.

I know the concept of toxins is not exactly how doctors and pharmacists look at prescription drugs, but the use of these products can cause major side effects by elimination of vitamins and minerals that our bodies need to allow enzyme reactions to work. There are thousands of these reactions needed to keep us alive. Some of the nutrient depletions are as follows:

Statin drugs deplete CoQ10, beta carotene, B vitamins, magnesium, calcium, zinc phosphorus, vitamin A

Diuretics deplete B1, magnesium, calcium and potassium

Oral contraceptives deplete beta carotene, B1, B2, B3, B6, B12, folic acid, biotin, vitamin C, magnesium, zinc, tryptophan and tyrosine

SSRI's deplete B6, B12, folic acid, vitamin D and sodium

Antidiabetics deplete CoQ10, folic acid and B12

Antibiotics deplete intestinal flora, biotin, inositol, B1, B2, B3, B12 and vitamin K

Proton pump inhibitors decrease stomach acid which depletes protein digestion and effects amino acid creation, neurotransmitters and doesn't process minerals

Female hormones such as oral contraceptives or hormone replacement therapy such as Premarin, Yaz, Mircette and Ortho-Tri-Cyclen deplete beneficial flora, DHEA, Folate, Magnesium, Melatonin,

Riboflavin, Selenium, Thiamin, Vitamin A, B5, B6, B12, C, and Zinc, (Taken from Dr. Isabella Wentz Hashimoto's Thyroiditis blog)

Many people are on more than one drug. They may be on four, five or ten drugs. These have many complicated pathways to follow in the body to work well.

They will eliminate vitamins and minerals. In combination with other drugs we are not able to estimate the level of malnutrition they are causing. Now add over the counter drugs to the heap. And, now let the patient take an acid inhibitor.

With minimal or no stomach acid how can we digest foods, digest medicines and protect against bugs and critters that need to be stopped with stomach acids?

It really doesn't help people to return to good health when the medical and pharmacologists forget the physiology of the body.

As a side note, many people taking prescription and over the counter drugs get rid of product by flushing them down the toilet. So now they wind up in our water supply. Our water companies do not remove these elements from our drinking or bathing water supply. Of course, these drugs are now in a less potent form, but there may be thousands and thousands of them in minute quantities, but they are still there. How do these affect a fetus, a newborn, a toddler, a teenager or a young adult? We have no studies to show the effect. But I think they do have a negative effect by starting nutrient depletions at a very early age and then the effect is compounded over years.

Drug-Induced Nutrient Depletions

- Female Hormones   FA, B6, B1, B3, B12, C, Mg, Zn
- Anticonvulsants: D, K, FA, Ca
- Anti-diabetic Drugs: CoQ10, B12
- Anti-hypertensives: B6, CoQ10, Ca, Mg, K, Zn
- Anti-inflammatory: Ca, K, Zn, Fe, B6, C, D, FA, K
- Cholesterol-lowering: CoQ10
- Beta-blockers: CoQ10, melatonin
- Phenothiazines/Tricyclics   B2, CoQ10
- Benzodiazepines: Melatonin
- Anti-ulcer medications: B12, FA, D, Ca, Fe, Zn, Protein
- Antibiotics: B-vitamins, vitamin K

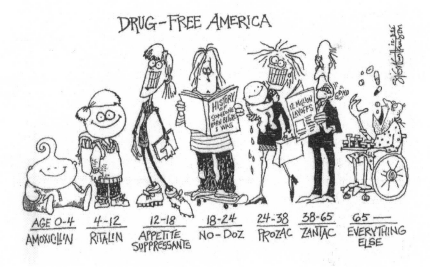

Chapter 5 - Pollutants

Many researches have determined that there are pollutants in our air, in our water supply, and in our food supply that can be the cause of disease conditions and stress and inflammation.

These pollutants lodge in our organs. They can affect our immune system and other systems, leading to inflammation which leads to diseases like auto immune diseases such as arthritis, diabetes, lupus, multiple sclerosis, Crohn's Disease, fibromyalgia, chronic fatigue, atherosclerosis, cancer, leukemia, lymphoma, and other chronic infections.

There are researchers that say that our genes are an important predictor of our future health, but more important is the environment, the epigenetics, that really affect our genes.

The question to be asked is what effect are the chemical toxins doing to us? There are thousands and thousands of chemical toxins. And there are thousands of environmental pesticides that wind up in our foods and in the air and in our water supply.

Are we benefiting from these toxins in the long run or are we slowly becoming sicker and sicker?

Dormant Viruses:

Recently I heard an ad on TV from a pharmaceutical company stating that the Hep C viruses need to be checked for in all people because it may be lying dormant in your body.

The key word is "dormant". What else is dormant? What about the dormant bacteria, viruses, molds and parasites? What about the dormant chemical toxins that are not found until disease conditions are manifested? How many years does it take to create a disease condition?

Blood and urine lab tests can't test for that. They can't test for those issues. Wow, can you see the rise in cost for tests that look for dormant states of all bacteria, viruses, parasites and even molds.

That's where the biofeedback can treat and assist to see the sensitivities of these critters. Let's catch the cause of a problem before it becomes a problem.

Chapter 6 - Biofeedback

"You never change things by fighting the existing reality. To change something, build a new model that makes the existing model obsolete."

— R. Buckminster Fuller

With the help of the biofeedback system we can look at sensitivities of viruses, fungus, mold, or bacteria or environmental chemicals before full blown disease, like cancer, becomes evident.

The use of herbs, as well as other supplements and homeopathy, can be evaluated and used as a treatment in the earlier stages of the disease or even before the disease is even determined.

Let's catch the problem of diseases before the disease even starts. Learn what your body needs to stay healthy, live better and live longer.

The mechanism of the biofeedback is a non-invasive computer system that "talks" to your body and records the response from the limbic system and skin responses. Sensitivities are recorded to different items tested and stress conditions are documented.

Biofeedback is a tool available to see what help the body needs to improve its state of health. In functional medicine, we don't look at symptoms of disease, rather we look at the cause of a disease and address that issue. The body will respond to that and get well. The item to balance a weakness in the body could be a single, or a group of vitamins, minerals, herbs, or homeopathic remedies.

The concept of homeopathy was a development of Dr. Hahnemann in 1796. The basis was that products of high energy levels can be used to cure like conditions.

Doctors of the day were using homeopathy and hospitals were using and teaching the concept of homeopathy. What a concept! Homeopathy works on the same principal as vaccinations do.

"Like treats like conditions" and builds immune responses with none of the side effects of most vaccines. The concept of homeopathy became out of favor due to ease of development and inexpensive cost of products. Today there are many practitioners that still understand and use the homeopathic concept.

We are all individuals and should be viewed as such. Different genetics and different blood types can have different reactions to drugs and to foods, vitamins, minerals, herbs and homeopathies.

What may be good food for me may not be good for you. Lab results have large ranges from low to high and what is really a good number for you? Does it represent the optimum physiologic value for that individual?

Biofeedback Expanded:

"You will observe with concern how long a useful truth may be known and exist, before it is generally received and practiced on."

Benjamin Franklin

The biofeedback system can check sensitivity to bacterial, viral, mold, fungal, environmental and pesticide conditions and the system can rebalance the body with homeopathic remedies, supplements, herbals, vitamins and minerals.

The biofeedback system can test for environmental issues, chemical toxins, heavy metals and mold and parasite sensitivities and food sensitivities. It does sound like a Star Trek medical recorder at an early stage of development.

The testing of these toxins is not difficult. Since they are not tested as a normal laboratory request, they are tested with the biofeedback as a normal protocol since better safe than sorry is a good rule to follow.

When the body says yes to questions asked by the bio-feedback system, we may get a better understanding of what the body needs to stay well, disease free and age gracefully. Emotions do have a major factor in how we feel, how we act and how healthy we are. Emotions can affect our physiology and can affect stress states which can increase inflammation and may even lead to disease conditions. Dr. Gabor Mate, in his book "When the Body Says No", summarizes "the latest scientific findings about the role that stress, and individual emotional makeup play in an array of diseases, including heart disease, diabetics, irritable bowel syndrome, multiple sclerosis, arthritis, cancer, ALS, among others."

Richard Earle, PhD states, "medical science searches high and low for the causes of cancer, MS, RA, CFS and a host of other conditions. One of the most pervasive factors leading to illness is the hidden stresses embedded in our daily lives. Stress can affect our immune defenses.

As you will see within this text, many stresses in our lives are discussed with the case studies. Stresses are shown by our individual patients and then we can see how they are balanced. The biofeedback system is a powerful tool to allow health practitioners to assist patients at a level never seen before. Balancing areas of stress is the first step to allow the body's immune system to work at freeing up immune defenses to attack more important disease states.

Superbugs:

The Scientific American issue of December 2016, has a very interesting article by Melinda Wenner Moyer entitled "The Looming Threat of Factory-Farm Superbugs."

Antibiotic-resistant bacteria from livestock, especially in pigs and chickens, pose a deadly risk to people. Nobody, especially the farm lobby, is doing anything to track or control the eminent danger. "Feed containing antibiotics are a necessity if they (the pigs) were to stay healthy in their crowded, manure-gilded home."

"Antibiotics seem to be transforming innocent farm animals into disease factories'

In the same article Dr. James Johnson, an infectious disease physician at the University of Minnesota states, "We have a long history of industries subverting public health." The article states the concern of researchers that the abundant use of antibiotics on farms is unraveling the medical community's ability to cure bacterial infections. "Stripped of the power of protective drugs, today's pedestrian health nuisances – ear infections, cuts, bronchitis – will become tomorrow's potential death sentences."

Livestock are given antibiotics for them to stay healthy and be a healthier source of food. They are given growth hormones to grow them faster and fatter for an earlier and better price at the market.

In addition to the antibiotics put in the animal feed, animal poop (manure) is used to fertilize crop fields too. This means that its bacteria and viruses and growth hormones and antibiotics are literally spread on the soil used to grow our food.

Manure from hog and dairy farms was applied to the soil and the number of antibiotic–resistant genes in the dirt went up four-fold in a 2016 study.

What are farmers, and corporate farms, doing to people's health? They can't be totally unaware of what they are creating in the guise of profit making. Can this be the cause of increases in poor health in people and animals? The Scientific American article certainly creates questions on the future of endangering public health due to increased uses of antibiotics in farm animals and using manure on produce.

Expand Causes of Diseases:

Let's expand the hypothesis of scientists who think that diseases are caused by viruses, bacteria, fungus and molds. Now we need to expand the list to include the toxins from chemicals, environmental pesticides, vaccines and our drinking water to the list. This is a scary list of toxins that affect everybody. I'm reminded of the witches in Macbeth adding things to the boiling cauldron. We are absorbing the toxins from the witch's brew.

So, let's go back to the earlier statement, or question, what is happening to our genetics when these epigenetic toxins are ingested?

We now have hundreds, if not thousands, of chemical insults affecting us daily. The question to ask is what happens to the offspring of the two folks who now combine all these chemical toxins? What about the second or fifth or tenth generation of offspring? Should we be concerned? Of course, we should. We should not wait till a disaster happens.

Underlying Cause of Disease:

We stated earlier that there are many doctors/researchers that state most diseases have an underlying cause.

These causes can be from bacteria, viruses, fungus, and molds. Can these come from our water supply? Can these invaders come from our food supply due to animal injections, vaccinations, food lots sprayed with pesticides?

No blood work or urine samples can pick up on any of these entities without specific and expensive tests.

The bio feedback system can detect these entities with levels of sensitivity testing and then balance these with herbs, anti-fungal, or homeopathic level remedies. The balancing steps use frequencies that are positive to each individual. When we balance a person, we look at the most basic and most essential vitamin, mineral, herb or homeopathic that will help obtain the best healing for the body. The newest fad of supplements may not be the product to use.

The question we ask is what the body is missing to achieve health and wellness.

Pre-Disease Conditions:

The process of evaluating pre-disease conditions with testing for chemical sensitivities, heavy metal toxicity, and viral, bacterial, fungal and parasitic entities can be tested and balanced with the bio-feedback system. What a great tool for the folks that are told they are well but do feel sick; or for those folks that are sick, and no medicine has helped them feel better.

Major Testing Areas:

The eight major areas of the bio-feedback system that can help people stay healthy are:

1.   Checking the nutrition that the body needs

2.   Checking the sensitivity to bacteria, viruses, mold, parasites

3.   Checking the sensitivity to chemicals, heavy metals and environmental toxins

4.   Checking acupuncture meridian points and systems

5.   Checking spinal nerve involvement

6.   Checking organ systems

7.   Checking health issues in the mouth

8.   Checking herbs, supplements and homeopathic products to balance sensitivities

To repeat, the steps used with the bio-communications system cover topics including acupuncture meridians, oral health, organ systems, food sensitivities, chemical sensitivities, heavy metal and environmental toxins, and also cover bacterial, viral, fungal and parasitic sensitivities and the health of your mouth.

What Is in The Food We Are Eating?

What is in the food we eat? This topic really got my attention. After listening to DVDs from the Institute for Brain Potential presented by M. Kuhn, RN, ND, and PhD. I thought a summary of the material would be of interest to everyone.

Dr. Kuhn's presentation about what is in the foods we eat expands to also talk about oil and gas fracking, toxins in hospitals, mercury in vaccinations and has you listening intently. I tried to abstract her teaching to bring to your attention the "stuff" we are eating. Another source is the book by Dr. Joseph Pizzorno *"The Toxin Solution"*.

What Toxins Surround Us?

I mentioned Rachel Carson's book, "Silent Spring" written over 50 years ago. When I read her book as a teenager I was intrigued about the uses of pesticides and the destruction on life and the environment. The effects were well stated by her in her book in 1962.

Well, we have taken environmental damage to further extremes since then. Dr. Kuhn's seminar expands on our latest environmental impacts. One of the latest books on this topic, "The Toxin Solution" by Dr. Joseph Pizzorno, discussed in detail how the toxic chemicals are affecting our health and what we can do to fix it. He discusses how hidden poisons in the air, water and food are destroying our health. His book covers many more statistics than I could provide. I have taken the toxin level further in the testing that I employ.

The reason the biofeedback system is needed to help you restore your health will be obvious after the discussion of the poisons and toxins we are exposed to in our daily lives.

There is not just one solution to the toxic problem. Since we are all individuals, we need to look at solutions designed for us. Consider the biofeedback as a gateway to balance sensitive issues years before disease conditions appear.

Inflammation as a Killer:

We all have brains that work 24 hours a day, for a lifetime. There are times we accept the advertisements that we see, what we hear and do not question what we are eating. We need to understand the quality of what we buy and eat to improve your life and health and to use complementary medicine to help achieve those goals.

Before we look at the stuff the food industry is feeding us, let's look at one of the killers in society today. The state of inflammation in our body is caused by injury, disease and by all the toxins we are ingesting.

A Time magazine cover story, Inflammation: The Secret Killer | Feb. 23, 2004, proclaimed that inflammation is a silent epidemic. It is a slow killer which can lead to many diseases.

We need to connect the inflammation and stress conditions with a way to balance the inflammation. Through balance our immune system should neutralize the toxins and then be ready to fight disease entities like viruses, bacteria, molds and parasites.

When an injury occurs to a tissue, whether it is from a bacterium, trauma, heat, cold, chemicals or other factors, multiple substances are released by the injured tissue. The entire complex of tissue changes is called inflammation. The body tries to "wall off" the spread of damaged tissues to aid in the healing process. In homeopathy, Dr. Reckeweg, in his concept of Homotoxicology, expanded the steps in which inflammation can cause damage to the cells and tissues. His descriptions show the progression of disease conditions as the level of inflammation intensifies. The longer the condition lasts the closer the cell and tissue approaches apoptosis (cell death).

Chapter 7 - Daily Living

The topic of importance is the normal life we live, the food we are eating, the air we are breathing, and the clothes we are wearing. Also, the place where we are sleeping, and the bathroom essentials we are using.

Earlier I mentioned fertilizers, vaccinations and pesticides. We are attacked daily by hormone infused produce and dairy, omega 6 rich products that are not in balance with omega 3 levels, indigestible fats that are trans fats, and poisons like arsenic, which is in the rice that we feed our babies and in baby foods, high fructose corn syrup, BPA chemically lined cans and lined aluminum bottles are attacking our health and immune systems.

When you think of rust on an old vehicle, back yard furniture or an old shovel, you are looking at a process called oxidation. This is when an oxygen molecule attaches to another chemical element and free radicals are created. This happens in our body every second. This is a "new" toxic element that our immune system needs to eliminate. If it is not eliminated this newly formed element can cause damage to our body.

A toxic element is formed that can attack our DNA and cause much damage and disease conditions, inflammation and organ stress from within our bodies. There are many ways to decrease the oxidative damage. There are diet books, exercise books and even antioxidant supplements to counteract free radicals. There are also foods. The wonderful world of colorful fruits and vegetables are a great first step in helping the body get rid of free radicals.

The usual first line of defense against cancer, for example, is chemotherapy and high dosages of direct radiation. Many are now looking at changes in diet and high nutritive means. When I found a cancer issue in my throat, with the biofeedback analysis, I referred myself to the ear, nose and throat center. After surgery, I had localized radiation treatment. During those sessions, I met with the dietitian and was amazed at the crazy diet she was proposing to the patients. It was reduced to a diet of sugar and more sugar. All the foods you should not eat were on the three-page document. I explained to her my background and recommended three cancer diet books for her to read. The medical oncologist listened to my suggestions, but no changes were made to their protocol.

The important vitamins to include in the diet are B-12, Vitamin E, folate, retinol, Vitamin C and carotenoids. The most important is beta carotene. The food sources are pumpkin, spinach, winter squash, carrots, avocados, cantaloupe, apricots and collard greens.

The group of minerals and trace elements are calcium, iodine, iron and selenium. There are other items to be used to fight cancer. "These include the allium compounds, dithiolthiones and isothiocyanates, terpenoids, phytoestrogens, flavonoids, phenolic compounds, protease inhibitors, phytic acid, glucosinolates and indoles, plant sterols, saponins, and chemicals found in various botanicals". More information can be found in the article by Dr. Jerrold J. Simon "Phytochemicals and Cancer," in the Nutritional Perspectives: Journal of the Council on Nutrition of the American Chiropractic Association, Vol. 40 No. 3.

Stress:

Stress is another insult on our bodies. There is the simple stress of having to get a specific project done on time. That is a stress that has a start and end date and is normally easily manageable. But the stress of a disease, a sick spouse, a sick child or a state of dying imposes a longer lasting stress which will create inflammation in the organs and the brain. This can lead to disease conditions.

Vaccinations

There has been much written about the safety of vaccinations. Do they cause autism, ADD, ADDH are questions that have been asked by many parents, doctors and scientists? Is a single vaccination the problem? Are the large quantities given to new born starting at two months the problem? What about the fact that the human immune systems take ten months to start to develop? There are many good books on the topic of vaccinations and here is a good place to mention the topic and the concerns.

A new vaccination controversy has come to our attention. Marisa Taylor of the Kaiser Health News published an article in The New Mexican, 8/4/17, stating "offshore human tests of herpes vaccine stir controversy". The article continues "defying U.S. safety protections for human trials, an American University and a group of wealthy libertarians, including a Donald Trump supporter, are backing the offshore testing of an experimental vaccine. Southern Illinois University and a research group are doing trials on the Caribbean Island of St. Kitts. Neither the Food and Drug Administration nor a safety panel known as the institutional review board, or IRB, monitored the testing of a vaccine its creators say prevent herpes outbreaks. "What they are doing is patently unethical" said Jonathan Zenilman, chief of John Hopkins Infectious Disease Division. "There is a reason why researchers rely on these protections. People can die." This type of offshore testing may be a future health hazard to watch out for. Again, politics and greed affect this approach to testing.

Toxins in our Lives:

The environment is another area that creates toxins which lead to stress and inflammation in the body. The environmental toxins are in:

The water we drink & the air we breathe

The foods we eat

The beauty products we put on our bodies

The household cleaning products we touch and smell

The drugs we ingest – pharmaceutical prescription and over the counter.

There are more than 100,000 chemicals used in manufacturing. There are more than 17,000 registered pesticides used in this country. When food is imported from other countries we may not be aware of the pesticides they use. Pesticides have been sprayed on foods, carried in the air and wind up in our water supplies.

They are used in agricultural farms, on golf courses, our gardens, our parks, in our schools, offices and playgrounds. And recently, instead of spraying the pesticides they are mixed with soil fertilizers that plants absorb into the cell wall of the plant, making it impossible to wash off.

There are chemicals used in our body care products, our soaps, and our detergents and in the processed foods we eat. Then add to that food colors, dyes and lots of preservatives. How can we be healthy? The list Dr. Kuhn presented of the dirty dozen of environmental toxins are the following:

• PCBs (polychlorinated biphenyls)
• Pesticides
• Mold/fungus

• Phthalates
• Volatile organic compounds
• Dioxin
• Asbestos
• Heavy metals
• Chloroform
• Chlorine and
• Fluoride, (which I added to the list).

The effects of these toxins are seen in human and wildlife since the 1960's. All the inflammation and pre-disease states we talk about for humans are in the pets we have and love. The "crappy" foods are mixed, dried, packaged and frozen and canned for our pets also.

Frequencies:

There are different frequencies around us every day. Radio and TV waves, WI FI, frequencies from the computers, hand held tablets, TV's, electric stoves, microwaves, power boxes outside our houses, frequencies from power lines, X-rays, the engine in your car and especially our cell phones.

Did you know that cell phones emit radiofrequency energy, called radio waves, which are a form of non-ionizing radiation? The tissues nearest to where the phone is held can absorb this energy. In the small print booklet that comes with the phone it says to keep the phone about 5/8 to 1 inch away from your ear. People keep phones in their bras, front or back pockets and sleep with them. This brings up questions of radiation to sex organs and other sensitive areas of the body. Can this cause brain damage? Is it carcinogenic?

What about microwave safety? This is an old topic of discussion and people forget quickly. Microwaves cause vitamins to be broken down into inactive substances. Microwaves can release potential toxic compounds from food packaging like plastic wraps, styrofoam containers and coffee cups.

Using the microwave to cook foods can result in a loss of antioxidant compounds and the nutritional value of protein is reduced. Breast milk warmed on high in the microwave will lose 96% of IgA which is needed for immunity of the baby.

Chapter 8 - Chemicals in & on our Food

The exposure of chemicals sprayed on our foods are toxic to our bodies. The burden of pesticides is underestimated by the medical community, the laboratories, and the government protection authorities and are toxic to our bodies in small amounts at a time but are stored up and then can be dangerous and even fatal.

The US has documented what pesticides can be used on our food products. Does that mean they are safe? Have they been tested for a substantial amount of time before they are released on society?

Already we are affecting the population of bees and butterflies Their population is down as much as 50%. The bees are needed to do the pollination of many of our food items. There is an interesting article in the March 2017 issue of Discover magazine titled Buzzkill, page 30, about the effect chemicals have on the bee population. The population of bees have decreased to a point that scientists are worried about how the needed fertilization of food products will continue.

The worldwide economy allows foods from other nations to be imported to this country and become part of the food choices we buy. Do those countries follow as strict guidelines on the use of pesticides and fertilizers as the US? None of these pesticides are listed on food labels.

Antibiotics:

There are many concerns about the massive uses of antibiotics in doctors' offices because bacteria have a way to develop "antibiotic resistance" very quickly. The part we normally do not think about is the huge quantity of antibiotics, like 80% produced in this country, are used on farm animals, foods given to the animals and on growing plants. These antibiotics wind up in the air, the water, and in the meat used as food. An interesting TED talk in 2015 by health author Maryn McKenna brings "Antibiotic Resistance" to the surface. The problem of antibiotic resistance is a definite concern to the medical community, the hospitals and to the CDC.

Radiation:

Who would think that radiation would affect our food and our food choices? The meltdown of the Fukishima reactors in Japan has created an environment that can last for decades. The air and water currents transmit radiation for thousands of miles and last for a long time. The waters off Japan have concentrations of radiation that will affect sea life for eons.

Fracking:

The other environmental issue is the retrieval of gas and oil contained in the ground miles beneath the surface. The technique used is called fracking. The process itself releases methane from the ground. The technique of fracking involves the infusion "frack fluids" which consist of many toxic chemicals to promote the process. Where do these chemicals go as they rise to the surface of the ground? They wind up in our water tables, in our drinking water, and in our house water which we use to wash our clothes, bath and cook with.

Drinking Water:

An important element in everyone's lives, our city drinking water, is contaminated with chemicals. What is in the water?

Let's begin with chlorine and fluoride. The chemical, or to be precise metal fluoride, was thought to contain tooth decay. Well, this is not the case. What it does do is create free radicals in the body and affects our endocrine system.

Chlorine is another chemical used to kill bacteria in the drinking water supply. It also affects the endocrine system and creates free radicals in the body. It would be much wiser to use Ozone to clean our water supply.

There are drugs, chlorine, fluoride and estrogens. Estrogens started to appear in the 1970's. There are more than 3,000 prescription drugs and more than 1,000 over the counter drugs that are toxins in our drinking water.

There is a total of more than 80,000 chemicals compounds that can be toxins in our drinking water supply. How could this be?

The next burden in the water supply is the thousands of prescription drugs and thousands of over the counter drugs that are flushed down the toilet and wind up in the drinking water supply.

There are thousands of other chemicals that flood our water supply from soaps, detergents, shampoos, hair dyes, clothing softeners, conditioners, tooth pastes, mouth washes and makeups. This creates some concoction of toxins.

The purchase of bottled water does not resolve elimination of these chemical toxins unless the water bottled was distilled or filtered with a reverse osmosis system. Most bottled water is taken from the city water supply. Very expensive tap water. And the bottled water does not have to state whether fluoride is in the water. The bottles never list the toxins contained in the bottle.

The recommendation is to filter your own water with a distiller or with a good filter and fill your own glass container. You will save lots of money and relieve the garbage dumps of plastic landslides.

Milk Products:

Are we being sold a bill of goods with many of the foods we eat? Let's look at milk and milk substitutes. I will not ask the question of why we drink milk from another species. But a glass of milk from a cow does have live bacteria and microorganisms which are beneficial to our growth and development.

But the government is not in favor of us drinking milk that has not been pasteurized, homogenized or even ultra- pasteurized. This sterilization creates a product that has no helpful organisms. The pasteurization kills vitamins, enzymes, antioxidants and bacteria.

Then the manufacturer adds vitamins and minerals which may not even be absorbable by our digestive system. The manufacturer has increased the levels of phosphate which can leach calcium from bones and create osteoporosis, cancer, colic, earaches and gut issues. The release of calcium can wind up in our blood vessels and cause cardiovascular disease.

When milk is ultra-pasteurized the texture is changed, and a product called Irish moss or red seaweed is added to improve the consistency. This product is carrageenan, which creates leaky gut in some people.

This allows food particles to enter the blood stream and excite the immune system.

Similar processing happens with milk drink replacements like soy, almonds and rice. They can be ultra-pasteurized, sweeteners added, carrageenan added, been thru a gassing process with propyl oxide (also known as antifreeze). They have been modified with GMO's or could have arsenic in the product. These are not mentioned on the labels.

Fermented Foods:

Some excellent food sources are fermented foods. Store bought products like sauerkraut have been pasteurized so there are no live organisms left that can help. Kimchee and sauerkraut need to be made at home to get the live cultures and benefits through fermentation. These cultures feed our gut bacteria. The bacteria are needed to created B and K vitamins, protect the gut wall, build immunoglobulins, improve digestion and help in the elimination process.

Healthy Gut Bacteria:

Since gut bacteria are so important to our health, please take probiotics, especially after taking antibiotics. Since antibiotics kill the gut bacteria we need to repopulate them as soon as possible. The gut bacteria will create more B and K vitamins, help digestion and build immunoglobulins.

What to look for in a probiotic? Are they to be kept cold or on a shelf? If the label says they were pasteurized, please do not buy! A probiotic needs food to keep them alive. This food is a fiber product that keeps them alive. It should be packaged in the probiotic's bottle and may be listed as a prebiotic or as a fiber.

Gluten Sensitivity:

And now we need to review other major concerns with our foods. We have all heard about gluten sensitivity. What is that? The wheat from decades ago is not the same wheat we are eating today. Today's wheat has been modified genetically and has improved the production for the farmer to sell more product all around the world. However, the

EU countries and Japan are not accepting the modified wheat. They are aware of the issues it is causing in the US.

There is a protein in the wheat called gliadin. This activates the opiate receptors in the brain which causes increased appetite. We have also modified the wheat with pesticides that have not been tested as safe. There is a term called protein glycation which increases inflammation, free radical production and oxidative stress. These are thought to increase the risk of dementia.

Other products that have been genetically modified are corn, sugar beets, and soy and canola beans. These genetic modifications are playing roulette with our health. Other countries do not want to take part in a game that may affect their health, or even affect the genetics of their offspring. We should not be a science experiment.

The GMO's product label does not need to show that the product has been modified. Only 100% organic means non-GMO. When rats are used as an experiment with the genetically modified foods, they grow tumors all through their bodies. These show up after the 90-day experiment and they are not included as part of the studies. The foods that are modified genetically are not exported to many world countries. The sad part of the scientific genetic modification experiment on us is the food industry does not need to label genetic modified products.

Animals eating GMO foods have also had an increase in diseases including tumors, birth defects and multiple organ damage. The milk industry, including dairy, uses a hormone called rBGH to increase milk production. This hormone is a synthetic version of BGH and is known to convert normal tissue into cancerous tissue.

Flame Retardants:

Flame retardants are used in drinks. The product BVO is a synthetic brominated vegetable oil. This alters the endocrine system and the central nervous system. The BVO causes skin rashes, acne, fatigue, loss of appetite and promotes iodine deficiencies. Thyroid conditions can also occur.

Food Additives:

Other additives to processed foods are more than 3,000 preservatives, flavors and colors. Red dye number 40, yellow dye number 5 and 7 and blue number 2 are harmful. These may lead to mental issues and behavioral problems. ADD or ADHD may occur. Refer to the Feingold Diet.

Shop Smart:

We need to be smart in the way we shop and in what foods we eat. There are no governmental agencies protecting us. We need to learn to search on the web and find some thoughtful organizations that are currently doing research for us. Reading labels is very important. There are times the label is so small you need a magnifying glass to read it. I joke with patients if you can't read the words or you can't eat the ingredient(s), don't buy the product.

We are in control of what we buy and what we eat or put on our body. The skin is a great absorber of products. Chemical toxins get absorbed through the skin quickly and wind up in our lymph and blood systems. Spend time to read labels and buy real foods. Spend time and read labels of beauty products and buy the product if you can eat it. That's right, if you eat the product, then put it on your body.

Storage Containers:

Do you know the hazards of food storage devices? There are designated numerical imprints on all plastic storage containers. Let's look at what is not safe to use.

PVC 3 is polyvinylchloride which is plastic wrap and is made into cooking oil bottles. PS 6 is polystyrene or Styrofoam, clear plastic containers which can leach styrene and is a human carcinogen. PC 7 is made of PBA and is used in microwaveable plastic containers, plastic ware and is used in baby bottles and as a lining in metal food containers.

The items #3, #6 and #7 are not healthy items to heat, freeze, and then defrost. All supermarket or sandwich items covered with plastic wraps should be rewrapped before refrigerating.

Use wraps #1, #2, #4, or #5 for safety. Do not use cling wrap. The bottom Styrofoam tray should be removed. Wax paper or butcher paper should be used. Styrofoam is also a product to be concerned about.

Heating with microwave is not recommended. Using the Styrofoam cup more than once is not recommended. The heat can leach styrene which is a potent carcinogen. Packages of frozen vegetables should not be heated in their plastic bags; turkeys in plastic bags should be removed from the bag before baking.

And what do we do with the millions of plastic water bottles? As you will see later, the biofeedback system can test for most of the chemicals and toxic elements. The fancy water bottles that sell vitamins, minerals, weight loss diets, and relaxation or energy waters are not a worthwhile benefit.

BPA:

Bisphenol A is in many consumer products like the fire-resistant makeup of clothing, sheets, blankets, pajamas, and in furniture stuffing and coverings. It is in the linings of food cans, soda cans, and coating of popcorn bags to stop microwave fires. It is in number 7 polycarbonate water bottles. It is in baby bottles and microwavable plastics.

When these are heated they release estrogens. The levels in all Americans are cause of concern due to the fact they are estrogen disruptors and may cause cellular damage.

Number 7 BPA increases prostate and breast cancer proliferation. Questions exist about the effect it has in the brain chemistry of the hippocampus, which is our memory center, and thus leading to dementia.

Some other thoughts and facts about BPA. During pregnancy does the high rate cause miscarriage? Does it cause autism, learning problems by age three, anxiety, allergies, and type two diabetes and low sperm counts?

BPA is a chemical used to firm plastic bottles. It has been shown to be a carcinogen. BPA is used to line cans and aluminum bottles that foods are stored in in the food stores. Teflon was to be removed from the pots and pans a few years ago. It is another carcinogen.

For cooking or storage use glass or stainless-steel containers. The safe plastics are Polyethylene #1 PETE for soft drinks and water bottles, #2 HDPE for milk and water bottles, #4 LDPE for wrapping films, baggies and grocery bags, and #5 PP for yogurt containers and syrup bottles. It is best to replace the old bad number plastics.

Another thought is if shopping for coffee filters do not use bleached filters. Manufactures use chemicals to make them white and the chemicals are in the coffee products we drink. Use the brown filters.

Fluorine:

An item in Time Magazine, 2/20/2017 was found to be of interest, "Fast Food Wrappers Could Be Toxic." A report in Environmental Science and Technology Letters found that about half of roughly 400 wrappers from 27 fast-food chain tested contained fluorine, a marker for the grease-resistant PFAS chemicals. Previous studies have linked PFAS exposure to thyroid issues, fertility problems, and increased risk of cancer, developmental delays, and other health issues."

FSS: Fat, Sweeteners, Seasonings:

Now let's talk about fats, sweeteners and seasonings. When we talk about fats it is important to remember that our brain is two thirds made up of fats. The fats act as an insulator that covers the branches of the neurons to allow electrical signals to transmit properly.

There are different types of fat. Cholesterol is an inflammatory fat. Saturated fats are solid at room temperatures and they are inflammatory. There are polyunsaturated fats. There are unsaturated fats which are liquid at room temperature. The mono fats are palm oil, palm kernel oil, canola oil, olive oil and coconut oil. The poly fats are omega 6 and are corn oil, sunflower seed oil, soybean oil and safflower oil. The anti-inflammatory oil is omega 3, fish oil, which is an essential oil and cannot be made by our body. The ratio of omega 6 to omega 3 is currently about 30 or 40 to 1. The good number should be 6 to 1 or even better 4 to 1. We know that olive oil is a good oil. When you purchase olive oil, read the label and make sure it is pure olive oil with no other oils added.

A list of which fats are:

Bad: omega 6 – canola, corn, vegetable; trans-fat, margarine and substitute butter which is made from chemicals.

Good: extra virgin olive, avocado, almond, hazelnut, flaxseed and walnut.

A point to emphasis is that most processed foods, or convenience foods, have a calculated salt, sugar and fat content to maximize taste appeal at a convenient, if not cheapest price. The sweeter the diet, the sweeter you want your food. The craving for salt is started at an early age. They are both addictive. By the way, sugar increases in the diet are associated with Alzheimer's disease.

Where is salt used? The list is long: breads, rolls, pizza, cold cuts and cured meats, poultry and chicken nuggets, canned soups and sandwiches. Salt is salt, whether it is table salt or sea salt. Think of herbal substitutes.

A sweetener to avoid is the so-called all-natural fruit sugar, High Fructose Corn Syrup (HFCS). This is made from corn starch.

Use organic cane sugar, stevia, organic raw honey, and organic maple syrup instead of HFCS. Other sugar substitutes in the different colored packets found on restaurant tables are not a good choice. They are known to decrease gut bacteria, can increase the likelihood of depression, may cause white blood cell cancer and may cause psychological disorders.

The non-sugar sweeteners are chemically modified to reduce calories. The coffee additives are chemically produced. Look at the labels and see if it is easy to read the list of ingredients. Sugars and sweeteners add flavor and taste to foods. The food manufacturer knows the correct amount of sweetener to affect your taste and create an addiction to make you eat more products. This is called a bliss point.

The product MSG is used to create better flavor and increase your appetite. MSG is a neurotoxin and creates hypertension and Dr. Blaylock discusses this in his book, "Neurotoxins that Kill". MSG can be in all foods. Looking for MSG as an ingredient on a label may not be an easy task. MSG is hidden by many different names. There are twenty or so different designations for MSG. It is in many foods, toothpaste, and mouthwash and in baby foods. Remember, MSG is used as a flavor enhancer, even in baby food. Cooks have known that food flavor enhancers will improve the taste of their foods. MSG is used to affect the hunger center in the hypothalamus and acts as a neurotransmitter killer – a neurotoxin. Please read the book *"Excitotoxins: The Taste That Kills"* by Dr. Blaylock.

There are food additives to make foods taste like raspberries or vanilla. They were taken from the rear glands of the beaver. And these are labeled as natural. The other issue is food dyes and colorings. These have been found to be carcinogenic. They are made from petrochemicals. Did you know that perfumes and toiletries are made to have longer lasting smells with the addition of petrochemicals? The other day I was about to buy salmon and in small letters the sign said artificially colored. With what? The salesclerk had no idea.

Inoculated Meats:

Beef, chicken, pork and fish have been inoculated with antibiotics or the feed they are eating in captivity have been genetically modified with pesticides or other chemicals to make them grow larger for the harvest. There is no information on the signs in the food market about the foods the animals have eaten. There are no signs about the antibiotics injected or placed in their food source. The best solution to this problem is to buy free range, cage free, wild source of meats. The natural state of the wild is important.

Pesticides on Crops:

Pesticides have been used on crops. Crops have been genetically modified with glyphosate or Roundup, or other scientific experiments that have not had years of medical discovery.

There is much written on the "horrific truth" about Roundup. Jeffrey Smith, author of "Seeds of Deception," says Monsanto is pretending that they are beneficial to the food and agriculture industry.

What they have is very, very dangerous. Dr. Seneff has stated that glyphosate is possibly "the most important factor in the development of multiple chronic diseases and conditions that have become prevalent in westernized societies." She states that two key problems are caused by glyphosate. One is nutritional deficiencies and the second is systemic toxicity. The diseases include allergies, cancer, Parkinson's disease, gastrointestinal diseases, harm to gut bacteria, obesity, depression, Alzheimer's disease, Multiple Sclerosis, autism, infertility, ALS and more.

Glyphosate is a systemic herbicide which is taken up by a plant and destroys many of the minerals of the plant and then we eat it. Studies have shown the chemical exposure to glyphosate is linked to obesity, learning disorders and infertility.

A recent news item on a new pesticide spray, dicamba, manufactured by Monsanto and BASF, drifted on neighboring farms and damaged millions of acres of unprotected soybeans and other crops in what is being called a man-made disaster. This was reported by Caitlin Dewey in the Washington Post and printed in the 8/30/17 issue of the New Mexican local paper. "Critics contend that the herbicide was approved by federal officials without enough data, particularly on the critical question of whether it could drift off target."

Sunscreen:

It is a sunny warm day and you apply sun screen to prevent sun burn. Well, you are applying titanium dioxide to your skin. It is a component of the metallic element titanium and is commonly used in paints, sunscreens and is added to hundreds of processed products to make them appear white. It is in coffee creamers, cake icing, and processed salad dressings.

Other Chemicals:

Titanium dioxide is used to whiten foods and coffee additives and lighteners. Potassium bromate is added to bread. This is a thyroid slowdown product. Arsenic is in rice and all rice products, especially in rice baby foods. Arsenic is in organic oatmeal. It can still be called organic!

Arsenic is used in wines to rid the liquid of its cloudy look. A protein put in bread is human hair called L-cysteine. Cheap and very available in the Far East. Children love mac and cheese. Look at the ingredients and you will find made from coal tar. Dyes are made from coal tars. Yellow #5, tartrazine, was linked to childhood hyperactivity in 2007.

The carcinogen trichloroethylene (TCE) is an industrial solvent that has leached into underground water sources near waste sites around the US. An article in the November 2017 issue of Scientific American discusses the "Poison-Eating Poplars" and the specialized bacteria helps trees clean up a superfund site. At three superfund sites the hybrid saplings were soaked in the bacteria and planted in the hazardous waste sites. In three years the trees lowered the surrounding TCE concentration below the EPA mandated drinking water limit.

Another health concern is acrylamide in foods. This toxin in food has the potential to increase the risk of developing cancer. The most important food groups contributing to acrylamide exposure are fried potato products, coffee, biscuits, crisp breads and soft breads. Acrylamide is a chemical that naturally forms in starchy food products during every-day high-temperature cooking (frying, baking, and roasting).

Cosmetics and Body Products:

The discussion of cosmetics can be lengthy. This is better living through chemistry. Toxicity abounds in these products. When you can't pronounce the words listed in the ingredients you know you are being fed more and more chemicals. A good website to become familiar with is www.safecosmetics.com.

Remember, toxins in become toxins out into our water supply after entering the sink and bath and toilet. They wind up in the water supply and it is unfiltered. These toxins are part of the end disrupters that we are drinking. They affect our hormones, our thyroid, and other glands even though they may be in parts per million. The affects are on adults and especially on children. Parabens are in most cosmetics. A great rule of thumb is if you can't feel safe eating it don't put it on your body. Your skin is a great absorption organ and chemicals will absorb to the lymph and blood systems quickly.

The article "Get Toxic Chemicals out of Cosmetics" by the editors of the November 2017 issue of Scientific American, states that laws are needed by the FDA to protect people. Their concern was the toxic chemical, lead acetate, which is a suspected neurotoxin, is used in hair dyes. Lead acetate has been banned for nearly a decade in Canada and Europe. The article, continues to list the chemicals found in shampoos and tooth paste. They state the US should protect its citizens, but studies of toxic substances are not made available by the manufacturers. The article states "at exposures typical of cosmetic users, several of these chemicals have been linked to cancer, impaired reproductive ability and compromised neurodevelopment in children." The article continues "consumers should not be forced to scrutinize the ingredient lists in their medicine cabinets and report adverse reactions. That should be the FDA's job."

Protection Agencies:

If you are frustrated with what you are reading you may ask who is protecting us from medical and chemical experimentation.

Well, there are some governmental agencies that are there to help us. FDA and EPA come to mind right away. But are they really concerned for us and our health or are they concerned with big business? If you are reading the latest news in 2017 you see changes in our protection happening every week. There is a seemingly constant rollback of many protection rules to help us stay healthy. These changes in rules effect oil drilling, pesticides, methane gas from wells, dumping chemicals in rivers and even climate change defenses.

We, the US, will no longer be a member of the world climate change group of 180 nations. It is sad our leaders are so enamored with their intelligence that they dismiss the science of world class scientist. Greed, stupidity and ignorance still are part of our society.

Diets:

"Let food be thy medicine and medicine be thy food" is the dictate from the ancient Greek physician Hippocrates.

My interest in diet is based on the how food affects the issues the patient is experiencing. I will suggest diets to minimize specific issues the patient is experiencing. My goal is to use foods that do not exacerbate health conditions and do not fight with the immune system. Remember, there is no one diet for everyone. We are individuals and we react to different foods differently. This is a high priority in working with patients.

I want the immune system to fight disease and not fight the foods you are eating. Since we are all individuals and of different genetic types, the same foods are not equally as good for each person. One must be aware of the reactions they are having to different foods. What food is good for me may cause a negative reaction like bloating for you. That is why diets do not fit all people. .No matter what diet I mention to my patients I always stress the importance of their reaction to specific food items. There are hundreds of diets that have been published and each has supporters. My feeling is that we should eat foods that do not create discomfort, bloating, gas or belching or restless nights of not sleeping. I like natural foods. I do not recommend processed foods that have no nutritional value. I use the biofeedback system to check the value of foods on an individual. The higher the better. The value of the food is your medicine.

In Europe there are warning labels about food dyes and additives. We are not as fortunate in the US. There are a few diets that specifically warn about food dyes and food coloring. Products like Jell-O have food dyes made from crude oils. The Feingold diet addresses the issues of foods, additives and hyperactivity.

We also don't address petrochemical additives to products like mouthwash, medicines, lipsticks, candies and lollypops. These artificial flavors have petroleum bases. Also, your lipstick may have lead in it.

Why would companies put silicon in food products? To save money. Look at nuggets, fresh or frozen. Red dyes in foods. Pills, mouth wash, toothpastes can be hazardous to your health. Propylene glycol is a preservative found in foods and hair and body beauty products and is found in anti-freeze.

It is used in foods to make biscuits, cakes, sweets and other baked goods. Spraying of pesticides on apples and other fruits can be hidden by the shellac that is sprayed over the pesticides. This is difficult to wash off the fruit.

The article by Mary Budinger *"The Ketogenic Revolution in Cancer"*, in the Townsend Letter August/September 2017 should be read by cancer physicians as well as dieticians, nutrition consultants and cancer patients. As a cancer patient I was given three sheets of diet information that was totally sugar based and totally wrong. I knew better and tried to educate the doctor and dietician to no avail. The ketogenic diet is regaining popularity with integrative cancer physicians.

Dr. Otto Warburg stated, "the prime cause of cancer is the replacement of the respiration of oxygen in normal body cells by fermentation of sugar". He was awarded the 1931 Nobel Prize in Physiology of Medicine for discovering how cells obtain energy from fermentation. The article states "the ketogenic strategy is designed to turn you from a sugar burner into a fat burner. If you are "in ketosis", you are burning fat, ketones. What patients eat is very low on carbohydrates, low on protein, and high in fat" A detailed description of the foods continues.

The biofeedback system does check food sensitivities. It can check over 400 food groups and list the foods that are "good" for you. There are specific diets that can be analyzed, and foods are suggested that are good for you.

In Chapter 13, Foods that are good for you, you'll find a few of the diets that can be followed. I do use Dr. Peter D'Adamo's "Diet for Your Blood Type", to highlight the list of good and/or bad foods and compare it to the foods listed and eliminate the foods that cause the patient any stress.

Why do we have nutrient depletion in our foods?

There are some factors in producing good quality foods. First is the soil the food is grown. Are the farmers using high quality soil with good fertilizers or are they using synthetic fertilizers and synthetic pesticides? Are the products organically grown? Are the soils depleted of nutrients due to the fact that the products are not following a rotation schedule? Are the products picked too early and before they are ripe? Are they refrigerated for months before made available for sale? How is the food processed? Is the food bleached? What synthetic vitamins are they adding to the foods? Are the synthetic vitamins useful to our body? Are synthetic vitamins made from petrochemicals in the laboratory?

Buy Local:

The best foods to eat would be to buy from local farmers to have the freshest fruit but not always the prettiest or shiniest. Travel time for shipping are at a minimum and growing time is increased which can improve the nutritional value of the food.

Another issue is what part of the world does our food come from? When you look at companies associated with other companies you see food being grown in the US but processed in other countries. Pork grown in the US is processed in China with poor conditions or chemical contaminants. Tuna may be grown or processed in other countries. Tilapia is grown in China with chicken farms above the ponds of Tilapia. The fish nourishment is feces and chicken foods.

Vegetables, like garlic, are grown overseas with fungicides, growth inhibitors animal and human feces as fertilizers and the final product is bleached in chlorine. And we buy these, eat these and are not aware of how they affect our health. Nowhere is this mentioned on the food labels.

Eating Healthy:

To eat healthy foods takes a lot of work. Read labels on everything. Buy foods from farmers markets, shop the perimeter of the supermarket, and avoid processed foods down the aisles. Imitation food is not good for any of us, especially our babies and young children. Eat real food and not too much. Read labels on everything that you eat, wear, place on your body and sit and sleep on. It demands some work, but the truth is you cannot trust the companies selling you products. They are businesses out to make money and may not be after your best interests. Better profits through chemistry should be the motto and not better living through chemistry.

Home Safety:

An important aspect of items affecting our health is in our homes. We are now aware of the dangers of the plastic balls of soap for use in washing machines. Little children think they are colorful items to play with and chew on and are poisoned. Softener sheets are great items to go into the mouths of kids.

Triclosan is a chemical used as an antimicrobial and preservative in hand washing solutions, detergents, deodorants, dental products, toothpaste, undergarments, children's toys, and in more than 140 different products and are endo-disruptors.

It is placed in foods and wines and affects the endocrine/thyroid function of all. It is found in water supplies, food sources and in urine samples. There are safer products on the market – green products. There are many unsafe, untested products in the supermarket.

Let's look at the chemicals in our furniture. The foam and pillow coverings in our couches are infused with flame retardants. Children chew the fabric and absorb those chemicals.

Our bedrooms are another source of concern. What do you sleep on? Fire retardants are in our mattresses, in our sheets and in our bedcoverings. Pajamas and nightgowns are laced with fire retardants. Other toxins are formaldehyde and triclosan.

Formaldehyde is in easy to care for permanent press sheets. It is in the glue of the box springs. Triclosan is used as an antibacterial in the bedding material and can cause inhalation issues, liver and thyroid problems. There are pesticides like arsenic in mattresses. These affect hormonal balances and increase cholesterol levels.

An important document I have patients complete is a 2-page Bio-Detoxification form to help aid me in understanding their level of toxins. The form is on the following two pages. The questions open many areas of a person's life, activities and involvements not normally remembered.

Complete Bio-Detoxification
Symptom Questionnaire

Rate each of the following symptoms based upon your typical health profile:

0 – Never or almost never have the symptoms
1 – Occasionally have it, effect is not severe
2 – Occasionally have it, effect is severe
3 – Frequently have it, effect is not severe
4 – Frequently have it, effect is severe

Digestive

Nausea or vomiting	
Diarrhea	
Constipation	
Bloated feeling	
Belching, passing gas	
Heartburn	
Total Score	

Emotions

Mood Swings	
Anxiety, fear, nervous	
Anger, irritability	
Depression	
Total Score	

Eyes

Watery, itchy eyes	
Swollen, reddened, sticky eyelids	
Dark circles under eyes	
Blurred, tunnel vision	
Total Score	

Lungs

Chest congestion	
Asthma, bronchitis	
Shortness of breath	
Difficulty breathing	
Total Score	

Weight

Binge eating/drinking	
Craving certain foods	
Excessive weight gain	
Compulsive eating	
Water retention	
Underweight	
Total Score	

Energy / Activity

Fatigue, sluggishness	
Apathy	
Hyperactivity	
Restlessness	
Total Score	

Head

Headaches	
Faintness	
Dizziness	
Insomnia	
Total Score	

Ears

Itchy ears	
Earaches, ear infections	
Drainage from ears	
Ringing in ears, hearing loss	
Total Score	

Mouth / Throat

Chronic Gagging	
Gagging, needing to clear throat	
Sore throat, hoarse	
Swollen or discolored tongue, gums or lips	
Canker sores	
Total Score	

Skin

Acne	
Hives, rashes, dry skin	
Hair loss	
Flushing, hot flashes	
Excessive sweating	
Total Score	

Joints / Muscles

Pain or aches in joints	
Arthritis	
Stiff, limited movement	
Pain, aches in muscles	
Weakness or tiredness	
Total Score	

Nose

Stuffy Nose	
Sinus problems	
Hay fever, allergies	
Sneezing attacks	
Excessive mucus	
Total Score	

Mind

Poor Memory	
Confusion	
Poor concentration	
Poor coordination	
Difficulty making decisions	
Stuttering, stammering	
Slurred speech	
Learning disabilities	
Total Score	

Other

Frequent illness	
Frequent, urgent urination	
Genital itch, discharge	
Total Score	

Total Score	

Add up the numbers to arrive at a total for each section. Then add the totals for each section to arrive at the grand total. If any individual section total is **10 or more**, or the grand total is **14 or more**, you may benefit from the **Complete Bio-Detoxification** program.

Pain & Toxicity Assessment

Yes - No *Mark the symptoms you experience:*

☐ ☐ Do you feel tired or fatigued?

☐ ☐ Do you experience early morning stiffness?

☐ ☐ Do you feel stiff after periods of rest?

☐ ☐ Do you feel dizzy, foggy-headed or have trouble concentrating?

☐ ☐ Do you experience cracking joints?

☐ ☐ Do you experience frequent back pain or headaches?

☐ ☐ Do you eat fast, fatty, processed or fried foods?

☐ ☐ Do you experience generalized aches and pains in the body?

☐ ☐ Do you experience frequent sinus problems?

☐ ☐ Do you use coffee, cigarettes, candy or soda to get "up"?

☐ ☐ Are you sleepy in the afternoon?

☐ ☐ Do you experience intestinal gas and bloating after meals?

☐ ☐ Do you bruise easily?

☐ ☐ Do you recover slowly from moderate exercise?

☐ ☐ Do you feel you don't exercise enough or feel sluggish and need to lose weight?

☐ ☐ Do you have food allergies, or are often exposed to chemicals, sedatives or stimulants?

☐ ☐ Do you take pain relievers to get rid of aches and pains?

☐ ☐ Do you have a family history of arthritis or auto-immune disorders?

☐ ☐ Do your bowels move less than twice per day?

☐ ☐ Are you working or living in a closed environment with exposure to fresh air less than twice a day?

☐ ☐ Do you use regular municipal water (non-filtered) for your shower?

☐ ☐ Do you purchase food from the "normal" section of the grocery store, instead of buying organic fresh foods?

☐ ☐ Do you change/replace the filter for the heating/air conditioning less than twice a year?

☐ ☐ Does the concept of trying a cleansing program to rid your body of toxins seem foreign to you?

_____ **Total your "Yes" and "No" answers**

If your **Yes score totals 4 or greater**, your current symptoms might be due to toxic overload and may suggest you need the **Complete BioDetoxification** program.

Chapter 9 - Dental Health

The next important area is dental health. The mouth is the most "dirty" part of the body. Most dentists do not explain the importance of dental cleanliness to patients. Brushing your teeth is important, but brushing your gums is extremely important. You will see from the next charts that the acupuncture meridian nerves are in the gums. Another topic not spoken about are the toxic ingredients in mouthwash, tooth paste, and any over the counter mouth drugs. Dyes, flavorings and polyurethane plastic abrasives to make teeth brighter can all be absorbed into our bodies or wind up in our drinking water as it is recycled. Another health issue is the toxic nature of fluoride. It is in many toothpastes as well as in many city water supplies.

The gut is the stomach and the intestines but also the mouth. What are some of the concerns in the mouth we should be aware of? An abscess in the gums is an inflamed bacterial infection. This can affect the nerve of the tooth. A root canal can affect the nerve root. A low-level infection can affect the nerve root. This may not seem of major importance, but when you look at the tooth/nerve chart you will see the level of relationship between your body's organs and emotional state and the tooth nerves. Other damage to the immune system can occur from dental surgery, removal of teeth, fluoride toxin, amalgam fillings and x-rays. An excellent review of dental health can be found on the web of Dr. Isabella Wentz, PharmD and in her books.

Tooth Chart:

The tooth numbering system is used to make you aware of the problems that can occur in your mouth. The numbering system refers to the nerves in the gum area above or below the tooth. The inflammation is in the nerve and gum tissue.

The tooth chart shows organ involvement and the second chart shows emotional involvement.

The biofeedback system can evaluate the stresses and helps to balance those stresses using nutritional, herbal and homeopathic remedies.

The tooth counting is the following:

69

Upper right starts number 1

Upper left is number 16

Lower left is number 17

Lower right is number 32

Tooth Nerve:

The importance of the tooth chart is not the tooth. It is the nerve innervation in the gums. Brushing your teeth is fine, but it is also important to brush your gums. The procedure is a very soft brush or the soft part of your finger.

The nerve is an acupuncture meridian nerve and it follows down to organs and down to your feet. Organ and emotional reactions can occur when the gums and nerves are inflamed. Heart, stomach digestion, thyroid, lungs, adrenals and kidneys can be affected with nerve inflammation. The chart "The Teeth and the Body" shows the right and left side of the body as columns. The horizontal table shows the joints, and the organs associated with the teeth/nerves involved.

The next chart shows emotional conditions, positive or negative, that can be a result of an inflamed nerve. Study the tooth chart and you will see the complexity of nerves, organs, diseases and emotions.

THE TEETH AND THE BODY
ENERGETIC INTER-RELATIONS

RIGHT SIDE					LEFT SIDE				

JOINTS

| Shoulder Elbow Sacro-iliac Hand Foot Toes | Jaw Hip Anterior knee | Shoulder Elbow Hand Foot Big toe | Posterior knee — Hip | Sacro-coccygeal Joint / Ankle joint | Sacro-coccygeal Joint / Ankle joint | Posterior knee — Hip | Shoulder Elbow Hand Foot Big toe | Jaw Hip Anterior knee | Shoulder Elbow Sacro-iliac Hand Foot Toes |

ORGANS

Ear	Tongue	Nose	Eye — Nose	Nose — Eye	Nose	Tongue	Ear
Heart	Pancreas	Lung	Liver — Kidney	Kidney — Liver	Lung	Spleen	Heart
Small intestine	Stomach Mammary gland	Large intestine	Gall bladder — Rectum Genito-urinary Prostate	Rectum Genito-urinary Prostate — Gall bladder	Large intestine	Stomach Mammary gland	Small intestine

TEETH

| Pituitary gland Ant. lobe | Para-Thyroid | Thyroid | Thymus | Pituitary gland Post. lobe | Pineal gland | Pineal gland | Pituitary gland Post. lobe | Thymus | Thyroid | Para-Thyroid | Pituitary gland Ant. lobe |

RIGHT

1	2	3	4	5	6	7	8	9	10	11	12	13	14	15	16

LEFT

32	31	30	29	28	27	26	25	24	23	22	21	20	19	18	17

RIGHT — LEFT

ORGANS

Small intestine — Ileo-cecal area	Large intestine	Stomach Mammary gland	Gall bladder — Adrenal gland Rectum Genito-urinary Prostate	Adrenal gland Rectum Genito-urinary Prostate — Gall bladder	Stomach Mammary gland	Large intestine	Small intestine
Heart	Lung	Pancreas	Liver — Kidney	Kidney — Liver	Spleen	Lung	Heart
Ear	Nose	Tongue	Eye — Nose	Nose — Eye	Tongue	Nose	Ear

JOINTS

| Shoulder Elbow Sacro-iliac Hand Foot Toes | Shoulder Elbow Hand Foot Big toe | Jaw Hip Anterior knee | Posterior knee — Hip | Sacro-coccygeal Joint / Ankle joint | Sacro-coccygeal Joint / Ankle joint | Hip — Jaw Hip Anterior knee | Shoulder Elbow Hand Foot Big toe | Shoulder Elbow Sacro-iliac Hand Foot Toes |

RIGHT SIDE					LEFT SIDE				

Chart developed by Dr. Voll and Dr. Kramer 1953   www.drwolfe.com

71

Tooth Chart

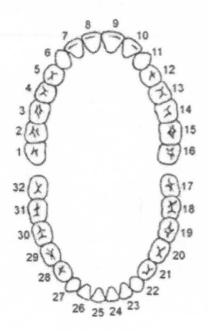

1. 3rd Molar (wisdom tooth)
2. 2nd Molar (12-yr molar)
3. 1st Molar (6-yr molar)
4. 2nd Bicuspid (2nd premolar)
5. 1st Bicuspid (1st premolar)
6. Cuspid (canine/eye tooth)
7. Lateral incisor
8. Central incisor
9. Central incisor
10. Lateral incisor
11. Cuspid (canine/eye tooth)
12. 1st Bicuspid (1st premolar)
13. 2nd Bicuspid (2nd premolar)
14. 1st Molar (6-yr molar)
15. 2nd Molar (12-yr molar)
16. 3rd Molar (wisdom tooth)
17. 3rd Molar (wisdom tooth)
18. 2nd Molar (12-yr molar)
19. 1st Molar (6-yr molar)
20. 2nd Bicuspid (2nd premolar)
21. 1st Bicuspid (1st premolar)
22. Cuspid (canine/eye tooth)
23. Lateral incisor
24. Central incisor
25. Central incisor
26. Lateral incisor
27. Cuspid (canine/eye tooth)
28. 1st Bicuspid (1st premolar)
29. 2nd Bicuspid (2nd premolar)
30. 1st Molar (6-yr molar)
31. 2nd Molar (12-yr molar)
32. 3rd Molar (wisdom tooth)

www.goodsamdental.org

TEETH - ORGANS	Positive Emotions	Negative Emotions
1 - Third Molar (top right) (Wisdom tooth) Heart, Duodenum	Joy Love Compassion	Rejection Resentment Family Problems
2 - Second Molar (top right) ORGANS Pancreas Stomach Bladder	Self-Esteem Order Security	Low Self-Esteem Depression Guilt Judgmental
3 - First Molar (top right) Liver, Kidneys Pancreas, Stomach	Determination Resolution Caring Humor	Anger Inflexibility Pride Disrespectful
4 - Second Premolar (top right) Right Lung, Large Intestine Small Intestine, Gall Bladder, Duodenum	Passion Determination Balance Ego	Monotony Possessiveness Revenge Critical
5 - First Premolar (top right) ORGANS Right Lung, Pancreas Large Intestine, Stomach	Excitement Purpose Self-Esteem Affection	Grief Condemnation Intolerance Love Pain
6 - Canine (top right) ORGAN Liver, Heart, Gall Bladder	Decisiveness Compassion Joy Pride	Anger Regret Family Problems Rejection
7 - Second Incisor (top right) ORGANS Right Kidney, Bladder, Urogenital	Caring Intimacy Order	Inflexibility Ego Problems Disorganized Aloof
8 - First Incisor (top right) ORGANS Right Kidney, Bladder, Urogenital	Clarity Acceptance Survival	Disrespect Emotional Outbursts Stubbornness
9 - First Incisor (top left) ORGANS Left Kidney, Bladder, Urogenital	Acceptance Intimacy Order	Inflexibility Ego Problems Survival Fear
10 - Second Incisor (top left) ORGANS Left Kidney, Bladder, Urogenital	Comforting Survival Closeness	Prideful Stubbornness Repression Avoidance of Intimacy

11 - Canine (top left) Liver, Heart, Bile Ducts	Resolution Purpose, Love Approval	Anger, Regret Sadness Resentment Critical
12 - First Premolar (top left) Left Lung, Liver, Pancreas Large Intestine, Stomach	Excitement Decisiveness Judgment Happiness	Grief Controlling Monotony Depression Spite
13 - Second Premolar (top left) Left Lung, Liver, Large Intestine Small Intestine, Gall Bladder, Duodenum	Enthusiasm Determination Balance Assimilation	Intolerance Negativity Fear Uneasiness Anti-social
14 - First Molar (top left) Liver, Kidneys, Spleen Stomach	Purpose Comforting Peace Affection	Self-Condemnation Regret Price Rejection Agitation
15 - Second Molar (top left) Spleen, Stomach, Bladder	Self-Love Calmness Security Closeness	Antagonism Emotional Conflict Lack of Self-love
16 - Third Molar (top left) (Wisdom tooth) Heart, Jejunum, Ileum	Compassion Joy Love	Avoidance Resentment Rejection
17 - Third Molar (bottom left) (Wisdom tooth) Heart, Liver, Jejunum	Joy Love Resolution Purpose	Depression Family Problems Guilt Regret
18 - Second Molar (bottom left) Pancreas Stomach Bladder	Passion Excitement Assimilation	Anger Grief Manipulative Self-centered
19 - First Molar (bottom left) Lung Large Intestine	Enthusiasm Balance Zest	Love Pain Controlling Revenge Over Critical
20 - Second Premolar (bottom left) Spleen Stomach	Peace Happiness Calmness	Condemnation Restless Agitation Emotional Conflicts

21 - First Premolar (bottom left) Spleen, Liver, Pancreas, Stomach	Self Love Enthusiasm Humor Security	Anger Lack of Self-love Resentment Regret
22 - Canine (bottom left) Liver, Lungs, Pancreas, Bile Ducts	Resolution Excitement Judgment	Resentment Disorganized Lack of Acceptance Over-bearing
23 - Second Incisor (bottom left) Left Kidney, Bladder Urogenital	Comforting Closeness Caring Order	Repression Pride Unhappy Sexual Feelings
24 - First Incisor (bottom right) Left Kidney, Bladder, Urogenital	Acceptance Intimacy Order	Inflexibility Anger Emotional Outbursts
25 - First Incisor (bottom right) Right Kidney, Bladder Urogenital	Clarity Acceptance Survival	Disrespect Stubbornness Sexual Problems
26 - Second Incisor (bottom right) Right Kidney, Bladder, Urogenital	Caring Intimacy Order	Disorganized Inflexible Disharmony
27 - Canine (bottom right) Liver, Lungs, Pancreas Gall Bladder	Judgment, Pride Decisiveness Compassion, Joy	Anger Regret Grief Condemnation Family Problems
28 - First Premolar (bottom right) Pancreas, Liver Stomach, Pylorus	Purpose Self-Esteem Affection	Judgmental, Insecurity Low Self-esteem Regretful
29 - Second Premolar (bottom right) Right Lung, Liver, Large Intestine Small Intestine, Gall Bladder, Duodenum	Passion Determination Balance Ego	Controlling Revenge, Unforgiving Manipulative Unyielding
30 - First Molar (bottom right) Large Intestine Ileocecal Region	Passion Balance Zest	Anti-social Pessimistic Grief Fear of the Future
31 - Second Molar (bottom right) Lung Large Intestine Ileocecal Region	Excitement Balance Passion	Depression Guilt Lack of Acceptance Negativity

32 - Third Molar (bottom right) (Wisdom tooth) Heart Ileum Ileocecal Region	Joy Love Compassion Approval	Family Problems Resentment Avoidance

Dr. Elmira Gadol - DMD
Holistic Dentistry
277 West End Ave #1C
New York, NY 10023
Phone: 212-501-7177
Fax: 646-657-0699
http://www.elmiragadol.com/

Sources:

Empirical Relationships Between Teeth, Organs, Disease Chart
Compiled by Thomas Rau, M.D.
Paracelsus Clinic, Lustmuhle, Switzerland

Using the tooth chart let's look at tooth number 1 in the right hand upper quadrant of the mouth. The nerve involvement could involve the ear, the small intestine, the heart, the hand, the foot and the toes, small intestine, the sacrum and pelvic joint (SI), and the anterior lobe of the pituitary.

Tooth number 32, is a mirror image of tooth 1 with the addition of the ileocecal area.

Following this path, it is fairly easy to read the nomenclature for all the teeth acupuncture meridian points.

The emotional aspect of each meridian is also explained as follows, tooth meridian 32 is joy, love, compassion and the need for approval.

The other tooth acupuncture involvements are easily followed.

Nerve Disease in Gums:

By following the nerve meridian of the teeth just look at all the organs and systems the nerves innervate.

Having periodontal issues and diseases is a way to affect organs in a negative way. Bacteria have a great place to hide in the mouth and can affect the nerves going to organs. Since the mouth is probably the most unclean part of our body, the suggestion is to put more time and skill brushing your teeth and don't forget brushing your tongue and gums with a soft tooth brush.

Chapter 10 - Not Feeling Well?

When you are not feeling well your medical doctor will send you for d laboratory blood and urine tests. Chemicals and pesticides are not tested for when we go to the lab for urine or blood work. These chemical and pesticides may the reason you are not feeling well or "just don't know why I'm not feeling right".

These are potent chemicals and are far from the thoughts of the physician and "normal" lab tests. The way to test for these toxins and inflammation and their generated stress is through biofeedback systems.

Your Body's Energy System:

Using your body's energetic system, the biofeedback system can provide information you are not normally aware of.

By placing your hand on the system's hand cradle the software will ask a series of questions, subconsciously, and receives your response subconsciously as a change in the electrical properties of your skin.

These scans are called biosurveys. The answers are recorded and analyzed by the computer software and reports are generated before and after analysis.

The biosurveys can include overall wellness, food sensitivities, organ system issues, nutritional needs, fungal, viral, bacterial and pesticide issues and other environmental issues. The system can evaluate heavy metal toxicity and chemical sensitivities and make suggestions for corrections. It can look at acupuncture meridian points and evaluate your dental health.

Remember many health problems begin in the mouth. The bacteria in your mouth can have profound conditions on your health and wellness.

Steps to Good Health:

The first session with a patient gathers information about their health history and their familial health history. An analysis is done to see if there are any environmental toxins. This can be multiple steps, to include heavy metals, chemicals, vaccinations, bacteria, viruses, mold/fungal and parasites. Food sensitivities are also checked for.

The goal is not for the body to fight food but to fight disease. The elimination of stresses to the body is done first to allow the body to be able to handle the proposed vitamins, minerals, herbs and homeopathic needed for the steps that will follow.

The next step is to look at other body sensitivities such as organs, teeth, digestion, cardiovascular, and gender specific issues including hormonal, neurological and nutritional deficiencies.

Knowing that not all products are good for everyone, the feedback system will analyze one or more supplements to see what is best for the patient to balance stresses that are out of range. It is a computerized test to determine the strength of a good vs. unfavorable supplement.

Pick the best that will do the most to correct a stress and inflamed condition. The approach that I like is to see what other areas of stress the nutritional item can affect. When a supplement states it will alter digestion the question to ask is what else does it affect? What else is in balance or not in balance?

Chapter 11 - Tests Used with Biofeedback

As an introduction to the biofeedback system, the following exhibits show tests for bacteria, viruses, heavy metals, chemicals, pesticides, water contaminants, molds and fungus and immune toxins. These will be explained in more detail with specific case studies presented later.

Water Contaminants:

The following two-page list shows a female patient age 62 with some health issues such as tiredness, anxiety at times, having sleep difficulty and experiencing joint and muscle pains.

She lives on a ranch and uses well water for bathing and cooking, but drinks purified bottled water. We muscle tested her well water along with city water from the tap, distilled water and reverse osmosis water. The well water was the weakest. We then ran a water contaminant biofeedback to see what chemicals she was stressed with. Her stress level was 9.9 and the list shows the chemicals she is stressed with and those her body could handle.

When a stress level is calculated by the biofeedback system, like 9.9, any number higher than an absolute 9.9 is considered a body stressor. Any number less than 9.9 means the body is able to handle that stress. When the body cannot handle a stress item it is necessary to develop a balancer to help the body handle that stress item.

Dr. Harold Steinberg, D.C.

Water Contaminants - The following is a list of water contaminants that can be tested. There are stress contaminants that are higher than 9.9 and are out of range and need to be balanced.

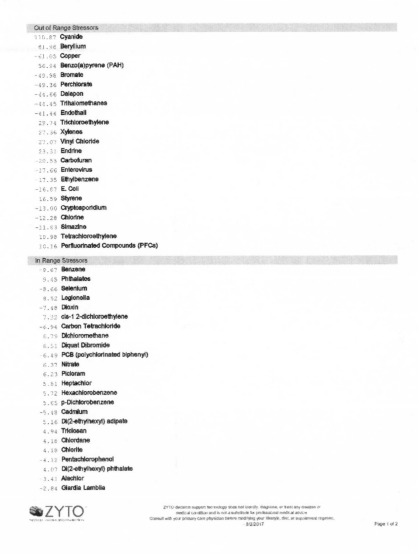

Out of Range Stressors

Value	Contaminant
116.87	Cyanide
81.98	Beryllium
-61.05	Copper
56.94	Benzo(a)pyrene (PAH)
-49.98	Bromate
-49.36	Perchlorate
-44.66	Dalapon
-44.45	Trihalomethanes
-41.44	Endothall
29.74	Trichloroethylene
27.36	Xylenes
27.07	Vinyl Chloride
23.31	Endrine
-20.53	Carbofuran
-17.66	Enterovirus
-17.35	Ethylbenzene
-16.87	E. Coli
16.59	Styrene
-13.00	Cryptosporidium
-12.28	Chlorine
-11.83	Simazine
10.98	Tetrachloroethylene
10.16	Perfluorinated Compounds (PFCs)

In Range Stressors

Value	Contaminant
-9.67	Benzene
9.45	Phthalates
-8.66	Selenium
8.52	Legionella
-7.48	Dioxin
7.22	cis-1 2-dichloroethylene
-6.94	Carbon Tetrachloride
6.79	Dichloromethane
6.51	Diquat Dibromide
6.49	PCB (polychlorinated biphenyl)
6.37	Nitrate
6.23	Picloram
5.81	Heptachlor
5.72	Hexachlorobenzene
5.65	p-Dichlorobenzene
-5.48	Cadmium
5.16	Di(2-ethylhexyl) adipate
4.94	Triclosan
4.18	Chlordane
4.19	Chlorite
-4.12	Pentachlorophenol
4.07	Di(2-ethylhexyl) phthalate
-3.41	Alachlor
-2.84	Giardia Lamblia

ZYTO

ZYTO decision support technology does not identify, diagnose, or treat any disease or medical condition and is not a substitute for professional medical advice. Consult with your primary care physician before modifying your lifestyle, diet, or supplement regimen.
8/2/2017

Page 1 of 2

82

Water Contaminants

2.80 trans-1 2-Dichloroethylene
2.79 Lindane
-2.71 1 2-Dichloroethane
-2.71 2,4-D
-2.29 Epichlorohydrin
-2.16 Glyphosate
-2.15 Haloacetic acids (HAA5)
-2.15 Radium 226 & 228
-2.14 Oxamyl
2.13 Mercury
-2.12 Hexachlorocyclopentadiene
-2.09 Beta Particles and Photon Emitters
2.07 Total Trihalomethanes (TTHMs)
-2.06 Antimony
-2.06 Toluene
2.04 1 2-Dibromo-3-chloropropane (DBCP)
2.03 1 1 1-Trichloroethane
1.42 Chromium
-1.41 Ethylene Dibromide
1.41 Hexavalent Chromium
1.39 Lead
1.38 Aluminum
-1.38 Asbestos
1.37 Radionuclides
-1.36 1 2-Dichloropropane
-1.36 Acrylamide
-1.35 1 2 4-Trichlorobenzene
-0.71 Fluoride
0.71 o-Dichlorobenzene
-0.70 Barium
-0.69 Arsenic
-0.69 Uranium
-0.68 1 1 2-Trichloroethane
-0.68 2 4 5-TP (Silvex)
0.00 Alpha Particles
0.00 Atrazine
0.00 Methoxychlor
0.00 Thallium

Dr. Harold Steinberg, D.C.

Bacteria:

The list below is some of the 330 bacteria that can be tested. In this example all are out of range to show the whole list of bacteria that can be tested.

Out of Range Stressors	
-36.21	Aerobacter Aerogenes Nos.
34.81	Haemophilus Influenza
31.56	Actinobacillus Actin.
28.77	Bacteroides spp.
28.21	Bac Friedlanderi
28.09	Angina Plaut Vin
-26.46	Streptococcus Hemolyains
26.25	Cat Scratch Disease
-24.35	Bacillus Faecalis Alkelingen.
23.83	Brucella Ovis
23.42	Bacteroides Oralis
22.79	Bacillus Morgan (Proteum Morgan)
-22.22	Camphylobacter Jejuni
22.08	Clostridium Sordellii
-21.57	Treponema Carateum
-21.31	Citrobacter Freundii
-21.22	Trench Mouth
-20.95	Mycobacterium Ulcerans
20.47	Staphylococcus Pneumonia
20.43	Mycobacterium Kansasii
-20.25	Pyrogenium Avis
-20.23	Tuberculinum Testicu
20.13	Salmonella Enteritidis
-19.93	Borrelia Novyi
-19.76	Pasturella
-19.74	Enterococcinum
19.49	Pyrogenium
19.38	Actinomycetemcomitans
19.31	Mycobacterium Scrofulaceum
18.99	Chlamydia Oculogenitalis
18.92	Camphylobacter Fetus
-18.88	Toxic Shock Syndrome Nos
-18.86	Bordetella Parapertussis
-18.49	Aeromonas Hydrophila
-17.66	Cholera (Vibrio Comma)
17.37	Rochalimaca Quintana
17.32	Tularemia
16.82	Hemprhagic Colitis
-16.75	Tuberculinum Burnett Nos.
16.55	L-Forms of Bacteria
-16.46	Clostridium Tertium
16.36	Bacillus Anthracis
16.35	Staphylococcus Aureus
16.12	Bartonella Bacilliformis
-15.61	Enterobacter
-15.55	Bejel
15.51	Legionella Micdadei
15.41	Clostridium Welchii, D type
15.32	Rickettsia Rickettsia

Bacteria

9.62 Meningococcinum Nos
9.53 Branhamella Ovis
-9.51 Pneumococcinum
9.48 Acute Bacterial Otitis
-9.46 Branhamella Cuniculi
9.40 Clostridium Bifermentans
9.28 Alcaligenes Faecalis
9.28 Anthrachinum
9.23 Clostridium Sporogenes
9.17 Anaerobic Gram-Positive Cocci (Peptostreptococcus)
-9.03 Diptheria Bacillus
-8.98 Bacillus Coli
-8.98 Cat Scratch Fever
-8.76 Bacillus Acidophilus (Lactobacillus)
8.76 Bacillus Gaertner (Salmon. Ent.)
8.76 Bacillus Pyocyaneus (Pseudomonas)
8.63 Enteropathogenic E Coli
-8.60 Streptococcus Rheumaticus
8.59 Bacteroides Fragilis
-8.49 Vibrio cholerae
8.43 Pertussis
-8.36 Typhinum
-8.30 Pyrogenium Crustacea
8.25 Leptospira
-8.22 Ehrlichiosis
-8.17 E. Coli
8.12 Pasteurella Multocida
8.05 Mycobacterium Chelonei
-7.97 Bacteroides Thetaiotamicron
7.97 Clostridium Cadaveres
7.94 Branhamella Caviae
-7.88 Moraxella
-7.83 Luesinum
7.77 Borrelia Morganii
-7.72 Actinomaura Viridis
7.69 Actinomyces israelii -mf
-7.64 Clostridium Paraputrif
-7.62 Actinomyces viscosus
7.51 Streptococcus Pharyngitis
7.46 Tetanus Antitoxin
-7.31 Glomerulonephritis
7.03 Pyrogenium Suis
6.96 Bacillus Subtilis
-6.96 Scarlet Fever
-6.94 Rickettsia Typhi
6.90 Paratyphoidinum
-6.80 Yersinia Pestis (Y. Pestis)
-6.79 Congenital Syphilis
-6.79 Pneumococcal Pneumonia

Bacteria

-15.28 Clostridium Perfringens
-14.98 Acinetobacter Haemolyticus
14.56 Bamaloides
14.51 Bacteroides Vulgatus
14.35 Clostridium Fallax
14.24 Legionella Pneumophila
-14.19 Bacillus Cereus
14.19 Borrelia Tillae
-13.94 Bordetella Pertussis
-13.66 Caulobacter Vibroides
-13.66 Puerperal Sepsis
13.41 Mycobacterium Avium
-13.29 Distemperinu
13.29 Staphylococcus Enterotoxins
13.25 Klebsiella
-12.98 Thermibacterium Bifidus
-12.66 Staphylococcus Coag
-12.66 Borrelia
-12.47 Agrobacterium Tumefaciens
-12.35 Borrelia Kochii
-12.30 Corynebacterium Diph
12.27 Bacterial Meningitis
11.81 Staphylococcus Saprophyticus
-11.73 Chlamydophila Psittaci
-11.72 Mycobacterium Marinum
-11.54 Streptococcus Impetigo
-11.35 Shigella Dysenteriae, Flexneri, & Sonnei
11.21 Helicobacter Pylori
11.20 Brucella Nectomae
-11.14 Serratia
-11.10 Legionella Dumoffi
-10.86 Enteric Fevers
10.69 Bacillus Dysenteriae (Shiga K.)
10.41 Tetanus (Clostridium Tet)
-10.37 Tuberculinum (Kent)
-10.32 Infant Pneumonitis
10.31 Bacillus Lactis Aerogenes
10.16 Enterobacteriaceae
10.13 Staphlococcal Hemolysins
9.94 Hafnia
-9.90 Streptococcus Haemol
-9.85 Bacillus Plasmaticum
-9.81 Bacteroides Putredinus
9.71 Borrelia Certeri
-9.66 Plesiomones Shigeloides
-9.66 Rickettsia Prowakekii
-9.65 Acinetobacter
9.64 Borrelia Recurrentis
-9.64 Tuberculinum Nos.

Bacteria

-6.72 Vibrio Mimicus
6.71 Meningitis Nosode
-6.63 Legionella Bozemanii
6.57 Bacteroides Trichoides
-6.47 Coxiella Burneti
6.45 Borrelia Burgdorferi
6.40 Borrelia Parkeri
-6.40 Borrelia Venezuelensis
6.29 Borrelia Hermsii
6.29 Brucella Abortus (Bang)
6.29 Clostridium Tetani
-6.26 Cervicitis
-6.22 Clostridium Dificile
6.11 Tuberculinum (Koch)
6.07 Catarrhel Mixed Flora
6.01 Streptococcinum B He
5.89 Actinomyce Temcomitan
-5.85 Gonococcinum
-5.85 Treponema Pallidum
-5.74 Actinobacillus Mallei
-5.74 Actinomyces Neeslundii
-5.71 Actinomyces Bovis
5.61 Edwardsiella
-5.55 Haemophilus Influenzae Nos.
-5.53 Lepromatous Leprosy
-5.48 Bac Tetani
-5.43 Actinobacillus Hominis
-5.42 Proteus
5.37 Morganella
-5.37 Peptostreptococcus
5.33 Mycoplasma Pneumoniae -bn
5.32 Bacillunum
-5.16 Bacillus Welchii
-5.12 Bacteroides Funduliformis
-5.12 Vibrio Vulnificus
-5.12 Yersinia Pseudotuberculois
-5.10 Bacillus Miserlum
-5.04 Bacillus Proteus (Proteus Mirabilis)
-4.84 Borrelia Persica
-4.84 Borrelia Vincentii
4.84 Branhamella Catarrhalis
-4.82 Botulismus
-4.80 Bang (Brucella Abortus)
-4.78 Borrelia Burgdorferi (Lyme)

Dr. Harold Steinberg, D.C.

Viruses:

There are 40 viruses that can be checked by the system, some are shown below. All viruses are out of range to show what can be tested.

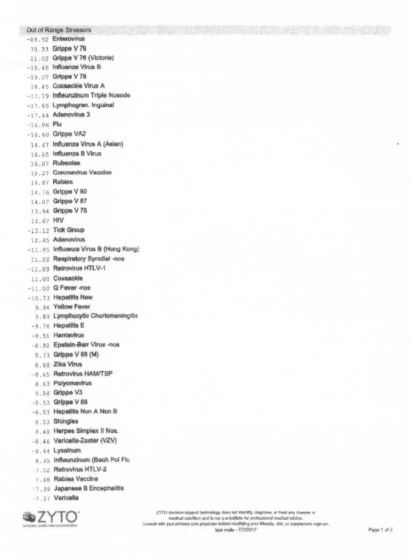

Out of Range Stressors	
~89.92	Enterovirus
70.33	Grippe V 79
21.02	Grippe V 76 (Victoria)
~19.48	Influenza Virus B
~19.07	Grippe V 78
18.45	Coxsackie Virus A
~17.79	Infleunzinum Triple Nosode
~17.65	Lymphogran. Inguinal
~17.44	Adenovirus 3
~16.86	Flu
~16.60	Grippe VA2
16.47	Influenza Virus A (Asian)
16.25	Influenza B Virus
16.07	Rubeolae
15.27	Coronevirus Vaccine
14.87	Rabies
14.76	Grippe V 80
14.07	Grippe V 87
13.94	Grippe V 75
13.67	HIV
~13.12	Tick Group
12.45	Adenovirus
~11.95	Influenza Virus B (Hong Kong)
11.22	Respiratory Synctial -nos
~11.09	Retrovirus HTLV-1
11.00	Coxsackie
~11.00	Q Fever -nos
~10.73	Hepatitis New
9.94	Yellow Fever
9.89	Lymphocytic Choriomeningitis
~9.78	Hepatitis E
~9.51	Hantavirus
~8.92	Epstein-Barr Virus -nos
8.73	Grippe V 86 (M)
8.68	Zika Virus
~8.65	Retrovirus HAM/TSP
8.63	Polyomavirus
8.58	Grippe V3
~8.53	Grippe V 88
~8.53	Hepatitis Non A Non B
8.53	Shingles
8.48	Herpes Simplex II Nos.
~8.46	Varicella-Zoster (VZV)
~8.44	Lyssinum
8.35	Infleunzinum (Bach Pol Flu
7.52	Retrovirus HTLV-2
7.48	Rabies Vaccine
~7.39	Japanese B Encephalitis
~7.37	Varicella

ZYTO

ZYTO decision-support technology does not identify, diagnose, or treat any disease or medical condition and is not a substitute for professional medical advice. Consult with your primary care physician before modifying your lifestyle, diet, or supplement regimen.
test male - 7/7/2017

Page 1 of 2

Viruses

7.33 Variolinum -nos
-7.21 Marburg
-7.14 Influencinum (Berlin 55)
-6.98 Adenovirus 39
-6.90 California Encephalitis La Crosse

Heavy Metals:

Heavy Metals can also be tested. The following are some of them.

-36.49 Thulium
-37.89 Iridium
-19.93 Tin
19.38 Holmium
17.88 Hafnium
-17.63 Titanium Dioxide
-17.13 Nickel -hm
-15.32 Calcium
11.85 Ethyl
11.53 Neodymium
-11.22 Tungsten
-10.84 Platinum
-10.54 Thorium
-10.37 Vanadium-hm
-9.92 Mercuric Salts
9.32 Lead-hm
-9.15 Lanthanum
8.91 Lutetium
7.83 Chromium
-7.23 Aluminum-hm
7.14 Barium
-6.73 Copper
-6.35 Antimony
5.93 Palladium -hm
-5.57 Gold
5.44 Manganese
-5.43 Methyl
5.41 Methyl Mercury
5.26 Cerium
-5.24 Tellurium
-5.18 Phenyl
5.18 Rhodium -hm
4.67 Thallium
4.64 Sodium Eathyl Mercuri
4.57 Potassium
4.45 Zinc-hm
-4.39 Zirconium
4.12 Niobium
3.67 Iron-hm
-3.51 Beryllium
-3.44 Dysprosium
-3.36 Mercury-hm
-3.35 Magnesium
-3.22 Gadolinium
-3.22 Germanium
2.74 Lithium
-2.69 Molybdenum
2.67 Osmium
-2.63 Yttrium

Heavy Metals

-2.61 Rubidium
-2.55 Uranium
-2.53 Titanium -hm

Chemicals:

Chemicals are another group of toxins to be tested.

Out of Range Stressors	
-42.31	Lead Iodide
23.85	Hexachlorophene
21.18	Acetylcholine Chlor
19.80	Succinic Acid
-19.68	Histidine - ch
19.65	Lead Chloride
-19.21	Temik
-17.85	Diethylstilbestrol
17.67	Xylene
17.63	Dioxin
-16.00	Rootox
15.51	Cleaning Supplies
-15.17	Lead Sulfate
14.88	Scrub Dessicant/ Stop Drop
-14.40	Gardrite/ Lawncare
-13.78	Nitric Acid
-13.75	Chloroform
13.36	Iodoform
-13.29	Comet Liquid
12.97	Zinc Cyanide
11.83	Lead Acetate
-11.34	Fantastic All Purpose Cleanser
-11.24	Ammonium Bromide
-11.14	Benzene
-10.98	Cleaner - Sodium Laural Sulfate
10.60	Pentachlorophenol
-10.53	Eosine
-10.42	Histamine
10.39	Varnishes
-10.31	Nylon
-10.25	Lead Phosphate
9.57	Mr. Clean
-9.41	Calcium Fluoride
9.36	Direct Mult-Purpose Cleaner
9.25	Ajax® Cleanser with Bleach
9.08	Gramozone
8.98	Nitroglycerin
8.90	Hydrogen Cyanide
-8.88	Grazone
8.18	Preeglone
-8.00	Soil Fume/ Borafuurneor
7.77	Ammonium Picrate
7.68	Ivomec
-7.67	Dieldrix/ Dieltrite
7.55	Lactic Acid
7.36	Citric Acid
7.29	Sentry Detergent/Disinfectant
-7.01	Paraffin
-6.98	Paint Thinner

Page 1 of 2

Chemicals

-6.95 Asulox
6.72 Malix/ Thiodan/ Thiofor
-6.35 Ammonium Iodide
-6.35 Cresol
6.30 Sorbic Acid
-6.29 Hydrazyne Iodide
6.27 Petroleum
6.26 Aniline
6.23 Tackle Cleaner Disinfectant
-6.22 Ammonium Valerate
6.12 Isoniazid
-5.65 Folimat
-5.56 Cleaner - Bleach
-5.56 Glyoxal
5.43 Top Job with Ammonia
-5.31 Phosphoric Acid
5.31 Triclosan
-5.22 Eosine B
4.85 Formic Acid
4.81 Ergot
4.77 Interferon
4.57 S.D.A.
4.52 Ripcord
4.47 Per 70 (Laundry Detergent)
-4.47 Resorcinol
4.46 Paint - oil based
-4.39 Oxaloacetic Acid
-4.37 Phenol
4.37 Pheyntoin
4.32 Tetrachloroethylene
-4.28 Touchweeder
-4.25 Magnesium Phosphate
4.25 Manganese Acetate
3.99 Calcium Phosphate
3.98 Baaudin/ Gesapon
3.97 Atax/ Control/ Scorpio/ Pyrox
-3.97 Ethanol
-3.96 Caprolactam

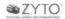

Dr. Harold Steinberg, D.C.

Pesticides:

Pesticides are another group that can be tested.

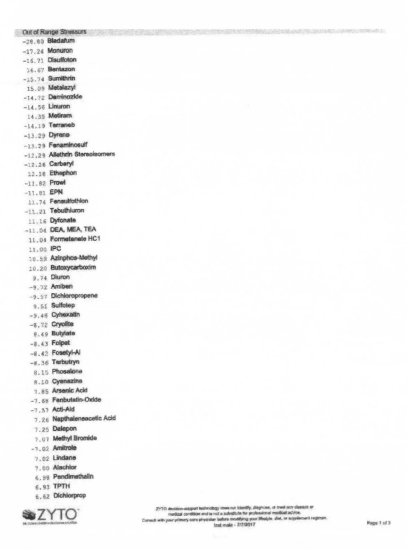

Out of Range Stressors	
-28.80	Bladafum
-17.24	Monuron
-16.71	Disulfoton
16.67	Bentazon
-15.74	Sumithrin
15.09	Metalaxyl
-14.72	Daminozide
-14.56	Linuron
14.35	Metiram
-14.19	Terraneb
-13.29	Dyrene
-13.29	Fenaminosulf
-12.28	Allethrin Stereoisomers
-12.26	Carbaryl
12.18	Ethephon
-11.82	Prowl
-11.81	EPN
11.74	Fensulfothion
-11.21	Tebuthiuron
11.16	Dyfonate
-11.04	DEA, MEA, TEA
11.04	Formetanate HC1
11.00	IPC
10.59	Azinphos-Methyl
10.20	Butoxycarboxim
9.74	Diuron
-9.72	Amiben
-9.57	Dichloropropene
9.51	Sulfotep
-9.46	Cyhexatin
-8.72	Cryolite
8.49	Butylate
-8.43	Folpet
-8.42	Fosetyl-Al
-8.36	Terbutryn
8.15	Phosalone
8.10	Cyanazine
7.85	Arsenic Acid
-7.68	Fenbutatin-Oxide
-7.57	Acti-Aid
7.26	Napthaleneacetic Acid
7.25	Dalapon
7.07	Methyl Bromide
-7.02	Amitrole
7.02	Lindane
7.00	Alachlor
6.99	Pendimethalin
6.93	TPTH
6.62	Dichlorprop

ZYTO

Pesticides

-6.42 Naled
-6.41 Demeton
-6.38 2,4-DP
6.31 Captan
-6.27 Amitraz
-6.26 Norflurazon
6.24 Captafol
-6.19 Methyl-Parathion
6.14 Zinc Phosphide
-6.12 MCPA
-6.09 Paraquat Dichloride
-5.96 Potassium Permanganate
5.96 Streptomycin
-5.84 Avitrol
5.71 Oxydemeton-Methyl
5.64 Carbofuran
5.64 Diallate
5.63 Nemacur
5.58 Chlordimeform HC1
-5.53 Nicotine (pesticide)
-5.50 Chlordane
5.46 Vikane
5.44 Methoxychlor
5.38 Warfarin
-5.36 2,4-DB
-5.16 Acti-Dione
-4.85 Oxytetracycline
4.81 DCPA
4.80 Chlorpyrifos
4.78 Dacthal
4.76 Diflubenzuron
-4.75 Dioxathion
-4.71 EPTC
4.69 Ethion
4.69 Sulfuryl Fluoride
-4.65 Fenthion
4.62 Sulprofos
-4.61 Aldrin
4.48 Boric Acid
4.21 2,4-D
4.14 Torak
-4.09 Aliette
4.05 DDT
4.02 Diazinon
4.01 Surflan
-3.99 Phosphamidon
3.99 Spike
-3.98 Metolachlor
-3.95 Diquat Dibromide

Page 2 of 3

Pesticides

3.89 Anilazine
3.89 Malathion
3.86 Fluchloralin
3.85 Metribuzin
3.49 Paarlan
3.47 Thiram
3.42 Trifluralin
3.36 Propargite
-3.33 Rotenone
-3.32 Phosmet
3.28 Aspon
-3.28 Basalin

Molds and Fungus:

Molds and Fungus can also be tested.

Out of Range Stressors	
34.55	Helminthosporium halodes
28.54	Mucor racemosus
-27.37	Dermatophilus congolensis
24.95	Sporothrix Schenckii
22.88	Lung Fungus
21.29	Mucor plumbeus
20.31	Agaricus muscarius -mf
-19.78	Skin & Nail Fungus
18.24	Trichophyton
-17.60	Rhodotorula Rubra
13.75	Deuteromycotina
12.68	Bermuda Grass Smut
-12.69	Claviceps
-12.57	Brain Fungus
11.17	Aspergillus flavus
-11.11	Johnson grass smut
-11.06	Fusarium
10.84	Barley Smut, Loose
-10.68	Corn Smut

Immune toxins

Immune toxins can be tested for stress levels.

Out of Range Stressors	
-39.88	Staphylococcinum
-28.44	Hepatitis B
-27.81	Respiratory Synctial Nos.
23.47	Epstein-Barr Virus
22.79	Meningococcinum
22.56	Catarrhal Mixed Flora
-19.13	Streptococcinum
18.72	Hepatitis A
-16.00	Tuberculinum Avis
-12.37	Coxsackie Virus B2
11.23	Cytomegalovirus Nos.
10.73	Coxsackie Virus B1
10.56	Legionella Pneumonphila
-9.92	Variolinum -nos

Balancing some of the above issues are shown with the following illustrations. The mechanism used is with the homeopathic concept of "like cures like"' The first step is to use the stressed item as a balancer and then make that item a homeopathic product and use them together as a balancer.

Looking at bacteria balancer below, we see the initial stress Bacteroides Fragilis at a 23.95 and Borrella Caucasica at 24.18. These were used as a balancer for the six items shown as a stressor. I used the system to create a homeopathic energetic remedy of the Bacteroides Fragilis at 32X and for the Borrella Caucasia at 200C. When the four balancer items are applied to the six stress items the second stress column shows they were brought into balance below the 5.95 level of the 4 individual items being tested.

Dr. Harold Steinberg, D.C.

In Range Stressors

-5.94 **Bacteroides Fragilis**
-4.93 **Pneumococcal Pneumonia**
-5.31 **Legionella Bozemanii**
 5.27 **Borrelia Caucasica**
 3.92 **Enteropathogenic E Coli**
 2.99 **Clostridium Tetani**

Balancers

 10.25 **Bacteroides Fragilis 32X**
 10.25 **Bacteroides Fragilis**
-24.18 **Borrelia Caucasica 200C**
-24.18 **Borrelia Caucasica**

The next illustration is of virus stressors. The Coxsackie virus A and Herpes Type VI were used as balancers with their energetic homeopathic 1000C and 70C levels. These four were used to balance the six shown viruses. The values of stress of the Coxsackie virus A went from a -26.51 down to 3.88 and the others went down below the 6.00 level to be balanced.

Dr. Harold Steinberg, D.C.

In Range Stressors

3.88 **Coxsackie Virus A**
-4.97 **Herpes Type VI**
-4.92 **Rabies**
-6.45 **Hepatitis Non A Non B**
4.43 **Influencinum (Berlin 55)**
5.54 **Grippe V 78**

Balancers

-26.51 **Coxsackie Virus A 1000C**
18.30 **Herpes Type VI 70C**
-26.51 **Coxsackie Virus A**
18.30 **Herpes Type VI**

Pesticides are shown in the next exhibit. The EPTC and Creosote items were used as the homeopathic remedies with their associated energetic homeopathic levels of 30X and 7X to bring the toxic range within balance. All were now below the level of 6 and in a range the body can balance the toxins.

Out of Range Stressors

In Range Stressors

    5.41 Fosetyl-Al
   -5.32 Dipropetryn
    4.02 Creosote
   -4.59 EPTC
   -4.34 Malathion
    4.16 Zinc Phosphide

Balancers

   31.00 EPTC 30X
  -28.56 Creosote 7X
   31.00 EPTC
  -28.56 Creosote

Chapter 12 - Case Studies

Case studies were done to show the type of testing that is used to determine the stresses a patient is having and how those were balanced. It is important to note that the studies are of actual patients, but I took the liberty to redact the patient's name and to also redact the products used in the study. The products are listed as Product A, Product B, Product C, Product D and Product E.

The philosophy of trying the least number of products that take care of the most stress conditions is my goal. Think of it as the 80/20 rule. Eighty percent of the stress is balanced by 20% of the products.

Case Study 1: Basic Reporting of the Biofeedback

Mrs. Y came in because she was not feeling well. At 58 years old she was tired and emotionally exhausted. She was given thyroid supplements but still felt run down. That was all the information she would tell me.

The results of the biofeedback showed organs that were stressed and listed recommended supplements for consideration. Her stress level is shown on the report titled "Organ VSI Results" at 7.04. The organs that are higher than the base number of 7.04 are the large intestines, liver, mammary glands, pancreas, pituitary and thyroid.

Since these are stressed areas a conversation was needed to understand if there are any issues she is aware of with her liver, mammary glands, pancreas, and thyroid.

The stress organs are the ones her body needs help balancing. Mrs. Y was interested in seeing how her next blood tests would compare to the reports produced by the biofeedback system before she started taking the recommended supplements.

A few weeks later we had the lab work to compare. The results were interesting. Based on the TSH her doctor reduced her thyroid medications. The doctor's interpretation was an over active thyroid.

That change didn't improve how she felt since her thyroid was actually underactive as shown by a thyroid stress of 11.29 shown on the chart. Her blood test also showed an increase of white blood cells.

Was leukemia part of her family history? Yes, it was, CLL could be the issue. She had had breast cancer and twenty lymph nodes were removed from her right axilla and a partially breast removal was done. That is why the mammary stress was high at a 16.92.

When the stress figures are over the average health numbers, it is a good place to have a discussion with the patient about the "why" of the numbers. Her liver was also stressed at 16.29. It could not convert T4 to T3. An iodine skin test was performed. Her energy level increased in a few hours. She is happy with the results and I put her on an iodine supplement.

Digestion was another issue as indicated by the stressed pancreas at 10.19. We discussed the foods she eats, and I asked what her blood type was. She didn't know. I did a blood type and she was an A. According to Dr. Peter D'Adamo's *"Eat for your Blood Type"* she should be a vegetarian with little animal meat. Her actual diet was meat protein based. I added HcL to her meals and the difference in her digestion was positive.

The acid reducing prescription and over the counter products suppress our own acid production. As you see from the list above the acid is needed to break down foods, especially proteins we eat. The normal reaction of the health care community is to write a script for an acid reducer when a patient complains about acid reflux. The problem is not too much acid, it is too little acid.

Because of low B12 the body can't produce enough stomach acid. Without stomach acid the body can't extract iron from food and B12 from food thus creating digestive problems and health problems since we need iron for carrying oxygen in our red blood cells and we need B12 for acid production and neurological balance. As you can see in the above chart there are many other vitamins and minerals that are not processed. Vitamin K is for blood clotting. Zinc is for our immune system.

The Vertebrae chart shows the involved nerves from the spine that are being stressed. The next chart, Teeth, shows the nerve meridians inflamed in her mouth. Looking at the tooth chart shows the possible organs and emotional involvement that could be experienced. The next chart is the TCM Meridians which shows the acupuncture meridians of the whole body that can be addressed by the acupuncturist she is seeing.

This example was used to show the basic testing that can be done with the biofeedback. Stresses can be from an incorrect diet or from a malfunctioning organ or the nerve innervation from acupuncture meridian points.

Dr. Harold Steinberg, D.C.

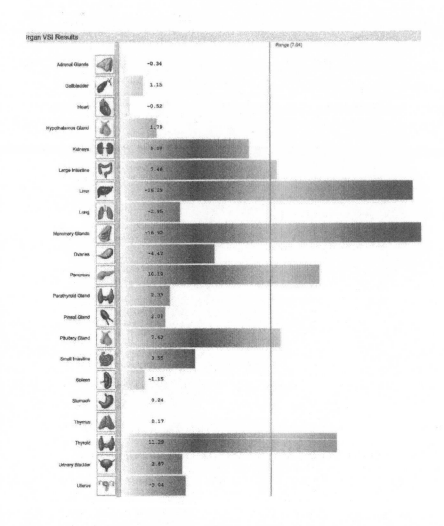

Toxic Overload

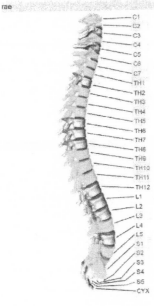

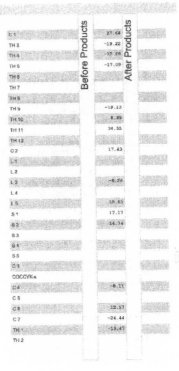

	Before Products	After Products
C 1	27.68	
TH 3	-19.22	
TH 4	-12.28	
TH 5	-17.09	
TH 6		
TH 7		
TH 8		
TH 9	-19.13	
TH 10	8.89	
TH 11	34.55	
TH 12		
C 2	17.43	
L 1		
L 2		
L 3	-8.26	
L 4		
L 5	15.65	
S 1	17.17	
S 2	14.74	
S 3		
S 4		
S 5		
C 3		
COCCYX-a		
C 4	-8.11	
C 5		
C 6	12.17	
C 7	-24.44	
TH 1	-19.47	
TH 2		

Dr. Harold Steinberg, D.C.

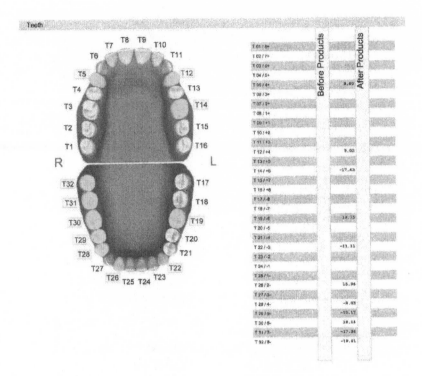

Teeth

Before Products	After Products
T 01 / 8+	
T 02 / 7+	
T 03 / 6+	
T 04 / 5+	
T 05 / 4+	9.99
T 06 / 3+	
T 07 / 2+	
T 08 / 1+	
T 09 / 1+	
T 10 / +2	
T 11 / +3	
T 12 / +4	9.03
T 13 / +5	
T 14 / +6	-17.43
T 15 / +7	
T 16 / +8	
T 17 / -8	
T 18 / -7	
T 19 / -6	18.75
T 20 / -5	
T 21 / -4	
T 22 / -3	-11.11
T 23 / -2	
T 24 / -1	
T 25 / 1-	
T 26 / 2-	15.96
T 27 / 3-	
T 28 / 4-	-9.03
T 29 / 5-	-15.17
T 30 / 6-	18.18
T 31 / 7-	-17.34
T 32 / 8-	-19.81

Toxic Overload

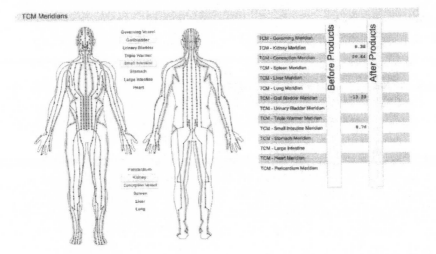

Case Study 2: Lyme, Bacteria, Virus, Mercury, Other Heavy Metals and Candida Toxins

Mrs. A is a 56-year-old female who travels to and from Central America multiple times a year. Her complaints were constant throat inflammation and heavy, deep coughing and exhaustion. She was dehydrated over two-week period and has been tired and stressed from the coughing. She also complained about a bladder infection. The biofeedback test showed a need for e-coli balance and a weakness in her heart. She said she gets bladder infections regularly. The biofeedback showed sensitivity to a large number of bacteria which were balanced by the nutritional supplements. Within two days her cough and exhaustion were eliminated. Another benefit was the E. coli was also balanced with cranberry juice and mannose and the urinary infection was eliminated.

The biofeedback Detox Focus Bio Survey results chart on the following page, showed paranasal and skin ranges beyond the stress level of 5.24. Her liver, joints and adrenal glands were on the stress side. The report results continue with an indication of sensitivity of Lyme at a level of 22.69. Mercury, heavy metals, bacteria, virus and candida were also elevated. Mrs. A did not remember being bit by a tick, but she was always hiking and around dogs while growing up. Detox Balancers/Foods to Avoid chart shows the foods to avoid strengthening her immune system. You would rather have your immune system fight disease than food items. Page 3 of the report shows the balancing of the products picked for her health improvement. Due to the many conditions involved it was necessary to recommend five different products to address all her conditions.

The" Balancer Results Comparison" report shows 32 items out of balance. When product A is applied 16 items were balanced. When product B is applied 13 items were balanced. Product C balanced 1 item. Product D balanced 1 item. The last product, E, balanced the last item.

Toxic Overload

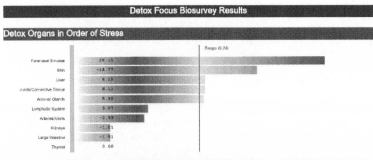

Detox Focus Biosurvey Results

Detox Organs in Order of Stress

Range (0-24)

Organ	Value
Paranasal Sinuses	26.15
Skin	14.77
Liver	6.15
Joints/Connective Tissue	6.11
Adrenal Glands	5.95
Lymphatic System	3.97
Arteries/Veins	2.93
Kidneys	1.51
Large Intestine	1.51
Thyroid	0.00

Detox Items in Order of Stress

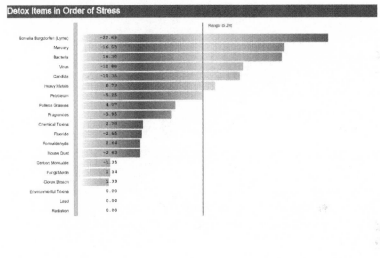

Range (0-24)

Item	Value
Borrelia Burgdorferi (Lyme)	22.43
Mercury	16.53
Bacteria	16.30
Virus	10.90
Candida	10.35
Heavy Metals	6.73
Petroleum	5.25
Pollens/Grasses	4.07
Fragrances	3.95
Chemical Toxins	2.70
Fluoride	2.65
Formaldehyde	2.64
House Dust	2.63
Carbon Monoxide	1.35
Fungi/Molds	1.34
Clorox Breach	1.33
Environmental Toxins	0.00
Lead	0.00
Radiation	0.00

113

Dr. Harold Steinberg, D.C.

Detox Balancers

Product A	1 Tablet 3 times per day
Product B	10 Drops 3 times per day
Product C	1 Tablet 1 times per day
Product D	1 Spray 3 times per day
Product E	10 Drops 3 times per day

Foods to Avoid

We tested 100 foods. These are the top foods you reacted to. The higher the number, the more stressing the food. Reaction numbers greater than 20 are higher reactive foods.
If the number is negative this food potentially makes you more tired. If the number is a high positive it can cause you to over-react, or be more stressed if eaten too often.
Look for food groups (dairy, grains, additives, sugars) or related foods (acid forming foods) in the list. Watch your reaction to the foods listed when you eat them again.

- 22.44 **Milk, Casein**
- 19.58 **Salmon**
- 17.60 **Olive Oil, Cold Pressed**
- 16.68 **Banana**
- 16.30 **Yogurt**
- 15.81 **Wine, White**
- -14.07 **Aspartame**
- -12.50 **Coffee**
- -12.18 **Grape (Red & Green)**
- -11.96 **Ketchup**
- 11.61 **Cheese, Swiss**
- -11.58 **Wheat, White Flour**
- -11.03 **Apple**
- 10.88 **Mustard**
- 10.86 **Yeast, Brewers**
- 10.83 **Lactose**
- 10.57 **FD&C Blue No.2**
- 10.41 **Egg, Yolk**
- 10.29 **Cheese, Mozzarella**
- 9.94 **Mushroom**

Toxic Overload

Balancer Results Comparison

	Baseline (32)	Product A (16)	Product B (3)	Product C (2)	Product D (1)	Product E (0)
Wine, White	15.81	8.54	10.05	20.67	14.39	
Skin	14.77	80.57	9.36	20.91		
Milk, Casein	22.44	15.99	5.37			
Aspartame	-14.07	-201.19				
Petroleum	-5.26	-8.27				
Banana	10.68	-30.94				
Heavy Metals	8.73	-18.33				
Coffee	-12.50	12.64				
Yogurt	10.30	11.86				
Virus	10.90	7.79				
Mushroom	9.94	7.88				
Bacteria	16.30	6.60				
Mercury	-18.53	-6.19				
Apple	-11.08	-5.76				
Salmon	10.58	-5.63				
Adrenal Glands	5.95	5.41				
Parasites, Sinuses	25.19					
Borrelia Burgdorferi (Lyme)	-22.59					
Olive Oil, Cold Pressed	17.60					
Grape (Red & Green)	-12.18					
Ketchup	-11.96					
Cheese, Swiss	11.61					
Wheat, White Flour	-11.56					
Mustard	10.88					
Yeast, Brewers	10.86					
Lactose	10.83					
FD&C Blue No 2	10.57					
Egg, Yolk	10.41					
Candida	-10.35					
Cheese, Mozzarella	10.29					
Liver	6.15					
Joints/Connective Tissue	6.11					

Case Study 3: Comprehensive Metabolism Study including Organ Stress, Internal and External Stressors

Mr. R is a 76-year-old retired scientist with a desire to lose weight and improve his performance in the gym. We accomplished both desires with a look at gender hormonal analysis and a weight loss recommendation product that helped burn sugar and let insulin do its job.

When I look at weight loss issues I like to see lab blood work. In this case it was not available.

The Organ Marker table shows stress level greater than 10.12 for his skin, joints, pancreas, heart and large intestines.

The following chart shows out of range top internal stressors which the system balanced with homeopathy remedies.

Mr. R does have difficulty going to sleep and has difficulty waking up without an alarm clock. Since cortisol and other hormones were on this list and was balanced we will evaluate the effect the balance has on his pancreas and his sleep issues. This makes him sluggish and keeps weight on.

The top stressors show pollens, penicillin, etc. which are balanced with homeopathic remedies. Positive thoughts are listed to help relaxation. The next charts include preferred food lists of fruits, vegetables, proteins and other foods. Each list shows positive foods and the bottom 5 items are foods to be avoided. The next chart shows 89 items out of balance. Product A balanced 60 items and product B balanced 25 and product C balanced 3 items. The last list shows all the items stressed and balanced.

Toxic Overload

Comprehensive Metabolism Scan

This innovative ZYTO decision support technology helps to discover information specific to your body's unique needs. We call this your biological preference. Using biocommunication, we are able to gather a vast amount of data about your body. This scan is a stimulus-response exchange between the software and your body. The responses generated by your body's energetic system provide valuable information at a level of which you are most likely not conscious.

Using this biocommunication technology you can discover specific, individualized information that will help design a personalized health and nutrition program specific to your body's needs. This individualized scan provides insights and information that can make a significant health difference.

Your Highest Organ Markers

This graph lists the top 5 most potentially stressed organ biomarkers. The higher the value the better probability that the organ many be in need of support. This technology does not diagnose or treat disease or illness, but gives you information on items that may be causing you excess stress.

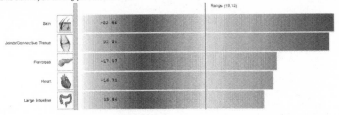

Spinal Stressors

Another factor in making sure your system is in balance is to make sure your vertebrae in your spine are aligned well. The next graph shows you the top 5 vertebrae that can use extra care right now.

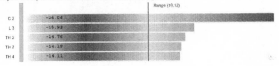

ZYTO decision-support technology does not identify, diagnose, or treat any disease or medical condition and is not a substitute for professional medical advice. Consult with your primary care physician before modifying your lifestyle, diet, or supplement regimen.
- 3/22/2017

Page 1 of 7

117

Dr. Harold Steinberg, D.C.

Our metabolism is controlled by internal and external factors. Internal factors such as hormones, neurotransmitters, along with nutritional imbalances can cause more stress on our system. This list shows you the top 10 metabolism factors to consider.

-56.31 **Epinephrine 4000X**
-42.89 **Aldosterone -hor 7X**
41.08 **Dopamine 30X**
32.03 **Cortisol -h 5X**
26.40 **Serotonin 30X**
22.15 **Norepinephrine 30X**
-21.39 **Iodine 4000X**
18.69 **Cholesterol 4000X**
17.19 **Biotin-vi 400X**
16.12 **Glucagon -h 10X**

Top External Stressors

Daily we are exposed to many external stress items like environmental pollutants, chemicals, heavy metals, bacteria, viral, fungal, and /or parasites. This list shows the top 10 external stress items for you. This does not mean you have these toxins in your system, just that your body overreacts to these stressors currently.

77.16 **Pollens Trees and Shrubs 3X**
69.88 **Penicillin 10X**
-67.15 **Pollens Flowers 3X**
58.67 **Trichloroethylene 30X**
56.35 **Pneumococcal Pneumonia 24X**
-56.17 **Cytomegalovirus Nos. 10X**
-55.00 **Leishmania Tropica 30X**
43.46 **Johnson grass smut 1000X**
38.77 **Pollens Grasses 100X**
-38.68 **Toxocara Cati 3X**

Positive Thinking Affirmations

Your thoughts create your feelings,
Your feelings create your actions,
Your actions create your results.

Change your thoughts - Change your life!

The following 3 statements resonant with your system currently. Repeat each statement a number of times out loud and notice the feelings that come up. Do they make you feel better? Use the statements that feel best to you as affirmations to receive what you desire.

I am safe and calm during the healing process
My body is healed, restored and filled with energy
I nurture my physical body in healthy and loving ways

Toxic Overload

Preferred Foods

One goal of metabolism balancing is to reduce inflammation caused by food reactions. Common foods that often cause inflammation are all types of sugar including fructose and fruit juice, artificial sweeteners, processed soy, gluten-based grains, genetically-modified corn, and dairy. We do not evaluate these potentially inflammatory foods as a preference for you.

We evaluated four categories of foods (Fruits, Vegetables, Proteins, and Other) to find out what you prefer in each category. The best or most preferred foods are at the top of the list, and the least preferred foods are at the bottom of the list. It is recommended to avoid the bottom 5 foods on each list.

Fruits

Banana
Apple
Grape (Red & Green)
Nectarine
Cantaloupe
Lime
Plum
Papaya
Mango
Raspberry
Cherry
Blueberry
Grapefruit
Lemon
Pineapple
Strawberry
Pear
Watermelon
Oranges
Honeydew Melon
Peach

Vegetables

Beet
Zucchini
Brussel Sprouts
Broccoli
Bean Sprouts
Pepper, Bell
Kale
Lettuce, Leaf
Carrot
Cucumber
String Bean (Green)
Onion
Spinach
Cabbage
Pea, Green
Tomato
Collard Greens
Lettuce, Romaine
Cauliflower
Asparagus

Celery

Proteins

Shrimp
Lobster
Beef
Perch
Halibut
Egg, Whole
Turkey, Dark Meat
Veal
Whitefish
Tilapia
Albacore
Turkey, White Meat
Codfish
Tuna Fish
Chicken, White Meat
Mutton (Lamb)
Salmon
Chicken, Dark Meat

Other Foods

Sunflower Seed
Psyllium Seed
Almond
Coconut Oil
Olive Oil
Coconut
Garbanzo Bean (Chickpeas)
Pinto Bean
Flax Seed
Cashew Nut
Almond Milk
Walnut, English
Black Bean
Rice, Brown
Avocado
Oat
Navy Bean (White)

Toxic Overload

Baseline
Biomarkers Out of Range: 89

Biomarkers Brought Into Range: 60
Category:
Usage Directions: 2 1/4 Milliliters 1 times per day

Additional BioMarkers Brought Into Range: 25
Category:

Additional BioMarkers Brought Into Range: 3
Category:

121

Dr. Harold Steinberg, D.C.

	Baseline (85)	Product A (29)	Product B (4)	Product C (1)	Product D (1)	Product E (1)
Methanol	23.86	13.16	12.93	-11.24	14.30	-22.24
Cytomegalovirus Nos.	-58.17	12.95	-19.70			
11-Deoxycortisol	-15.96	-21.69	14.37			
17a-Hydroxypregnenolone	-11.80	-13.89	10.31			
Epinephrine	-58.31	51.43				
Rubella Nos.	16.81	-30.06				
Power Lines	-14.57	29.94				
C 2	-26.04	-23.23				
Rhodotorula Rubra	14.24	21.26				
Toxocara Canis	15.92	-20.95				
Dog Hair	-22.12	-19.08				
Iron-fvm	-29.17	-17.63				
Penicillin	82.88	17.60				
Johnson grass smut	-43.45	-17.16				
TH 4	14.11	-16.41				
Ethyl	-14.42	16.06				
Bermuda Grass Smut	11.68	15.90				
E. Coli	-34.61	-14.40				
Klebsiella	-14.78	-13.11				
Rayon	12.89	-12.89				
Aldosterone mx	-42.64	-12.65				
Glyphosate	-19.34	12.53				
Potent Weeds	22.78	11.41				
Cholecystokinin	-14.35	11.24				
Agaricus muscarius -mf	33.47	-10.98				
Iodine	-21.39	-10.96				
Dioxin	-17.11	10.78				
Petroleum	15.63	10.89				
Pneumococcal Pneumonia	55.39	10.55				
Potens Trees and Shrubs	77.18					
Potens Flowers	47.18					
Trichloroethylene	56.67					
Leishmania Tropica	-56.90					
Dopamine	41.08					
Potenc Grasses	38.77					
Toxocara Cati	-38.88					
Nail Fungus	36.97					
Entamoeba Gingivalis	-32.25					
Cortisol -f	32.03					
Paragonimus Westermani	31.43					
Enterculus	28.64					
Cigarette Smoke	28.60					
Enterobius Verm (OX)	28.54					
Otitis Media Nos.	-27.82					
Mononucleosis, Infectious	26.74					
Serotonin	26.40					
Tuberculinum	-26.70					
Pertussin (Bordetella)	25.08					
DMDM Hydantoin & Urea (Imidazolidinyl)	-24.96					
Skin	22.86					

Toxic Overload

Joints/Connective Tissue	22.41
Norepinephrine	22.15
Epstein-Barr Virus	21.28
Paint Thinner	20.96
Mucor racemosus	19.76
Cell Phone	19.04
Toxoplasma Gondii Nos	18.98
Cholesterol	18.69
Aluminum	17.68
Potassium Iodide ch	17.60
Biotin-vi	17.19
Pancreas	17.07
Uranium	16.79
Clostridium Diffici	16.74
Heart	16.71
Glucagon -h	16.12
L 5	15.92
Large Intestine	15.86
Alcohol -dh	15.76
Lactic Acid	15.49
17a -Hydroxyprogesterone	15.47
Low Lipa	15.44
Adrenalin	15.23
TH 2	14.76
Lead	14.76
Dientamoeba Fragilis	14.59
TH 7	14.19
Silver	14.09
Cerium	13.97
Pregnenolone	13.36
Lung Fungus	13.26
Gold	12.79
Botulinum	12.05
Arsenic	11.68
Asbestos	11.53
Copper	11.52
Oxymetabacterium Anaerobius	11.46
T4 - Thyroxine	11.25
Acetylcholine Chloride	10.48

Case Study 4: Organ Stress, Candida, Bacteria, Lyme, Carbon Monoxide, Heavy Metals and Environmental Toxins

Mrs. J is a female aged 58 with anxiety issues due to work, family and divorced life. She is tired, and all her muscles hurt. She can't exercise and feels not able to complete her daily tasks.

The Organ Reaction chart shows her stress level as 3.21 as indicated by the line at the middle of the chart. The same chart lists CNS at 36.35 which is a high stress level in relation to 3.21. The adrenal glands are stressed at 10.70. The next chart shows the areas of electric/wireless stress at 8.26 and chemical toxins of 8.14.

The follow charts show lists of chemical toxins, electronic toxins, food reactions, immune toxins, molds, parasites and pesticide toxins.

The biofeedback system generated homeopathic remedies for the above list of toxins. These remedies together with four supplement balancers can assist Mrs. J's recovery process.

Toxic Overload

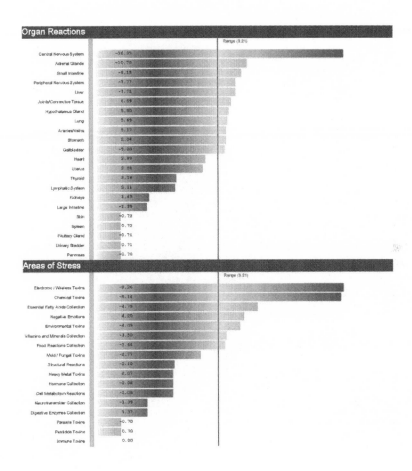

Organ Reactions

Range (3.21)

Central Nervous System	-36.35
Adrenal Glands	-10.70
Small Intestine	-8.15
Peripheral Nervous System	-7.77
Liver	-7.71
Joints/Connective Tissue	6.89
Hypothalamus Gland	5.80
Lung	5.69
Arteries/Veins	5.11
Stomach	5.04
Gallbladder	-5.00
Heart	2.89
Uterus	2.68
Thyroid	2.16
Lymphatic System	2.11
Kidneys	1.45
Large Intestine	-1.39
Skin	-0.72
Spleen	0.72
Pituitary Gland	-0.71
Urinary Bladder	0.71
Pancreas	-0.70

Areas of Stress

Range (3.21)

Electronic / Wireless Toxins	-9.26
Chemical Toxins	-8.14
Essential Fatty Acids Collection	-4.79
Negative Emotions	4.20
Environmental Toxins	-4.09
Vitamins and Minerals Collection	-3.50
Food Reactions Collection	-3.44
Mold / Fungal Toxins	-2.77
Structural Reactions	-2.15
Heavy Metal Toxins	2.07
Hormone Collection	-2.06
Cell Metabolism Reactions	-1.05
Neurotransmitter Collection	-1.39
Digestive Enzymes Collection	1.31
Parasite Toxins	-0.70
Pesticide Toxins	0.70
Immune Toxins	0.00

Dr. Harold Steinberg, D.C.

Top Items Out of Balance by Category

Chemical Toxins
- -39.06 Lysol Pine Action
- 27.83 Sodium Lauryl Sulfate or Sodium Laureth Sulfate
- -26.16 Salicylic Acid
- 15.69 Soft Scrub Cleanser
- 15.61 Trihalomethanes
- 13.08 Acetone
- -12.04 Potassium Iodide-ch
- 11.81 Trichloroethylene
- 10.61 Mercury
- 10.32 Lead

Electronic / Wireless Toxins
- -19.47 Alarm Clock
- -16.27 TV

Environmental Toxins
- -9.96 Rayon

Essential Fatty Acids Collection
- -12.19 Omega-3 (Linolenic Acid)

Food Reactions Collection
- -13.34 White Wine
- 13.66 Sunflower Oil
- 13.48 Superheated Vegetable Fat
- -13.23 Green Tea
- -13.21 BHA & BHT
- -13.00 Sweet & Low
- 10.71 2% Milk

Heavy Metal Toxins
- 15.94 Cadmium
- 15.10 Zirconium
- 11.97 Sodium Eethyl Mercuri
- 10.80 Uranium

Immune Toxins
- 38.88 Mycoplasma Pneumoniae
- 15.46 E. Coli

Mold / Fungal Toxins
- 17.55 Candida albican
- -12.46 Deuteromycotina
- 10.17 Agaricus muscarius -mf

Parasite Toxins
- 13.84 Taenia Solium

Pesticide Toxins
- -11.53 Metaldehyde
- -10.03 Chlordane

Vitamins and Minerals Collection
-12.05 **Zinc Oxide**
11.52 **Vitamin B5**

Dr. Harold Steinberg, D.C.

Balancers

36.91	Product A	1 Tablet 1 times per day
22.90	Product B	1 Tablet 1 times per day
18.77	Product C	1 Tablet 1 times per day
14.13	Product D	1 Tablet 1 times per day
11.73	Product E	

Potency Results on Stressors

- 10.71 **2% Milk 40X**
- 15.08 **Acetone 4000X**
- ~10.70 **Adrenal Glands 500X**
- 10.17 **Agaricus muscarius -mf 40X**
- -19.47 **Alarm Clock 4000X**
- 5.17 **Arteries/Veins 8X**
- -13.21 **BHA & BHT 100X**
- 15.94 **Cadmium 1X**
- 17.55 **Candida albican 500X**
- -2.05 **Cell Metabolism Reactions 4000X**
- -36.35 **Central Nervous System 40X**
- -8.14 **Chemical Toxins 5X**
- -10.03 **Chlordane 700X**
- -12.46 **Deuteromycotina 100X**
- 1.37 **Digestive Enzymes Collection 10X**
- 15.46 **E. Coli 400X**
- -8.26 **Electronic / Wireless Toxins 1000X**
- -4.09 **Environmental Toxins 500X**
- -4.79 **Essential Fatty Acids Collection 100X**
- -3.44 **Food Reactions Collection 5X**
- -5.00 **Gallbladder 700X**
- -13.23 **Green Tea 8X**
- 2.89 **Heart 24X**
- 2.07 **Heavy Metal Toxins 15X**
- -2.06 **Hormone Collection 30X**
- 5.60 **Hypothalamus Gland 3X**
- 0.00 **Immune Toxins 500X**
- 6.49 **Joints/Connective Tissue 5X**
- 1.43 **Kidneys 500X**
- -1.39 **Large Intestine 1X**
- 10.32 **Lead 10X**
- -7.71 **Liver 500X**
- 5.69 **Lung 3X**
- 2.11 **Lymphatic System 24X**
- -39.06 **Lysol Pine Action 1000X**
- 10.61 **Mercury 1000X**
- -11.53 **Metaldehyde 10X**
- -2.77 **Mold / Fungal Toxins 3X**
- 39.68 **Mycoplasma Pneumoniae 30X**
- 4.20 **Negative Emotions 40X**

-1.39 Neurotransmitter Collection 400X
-12.19 Omega-3 (Linolenic Acid) 8X
-0.70 Pancreas 4000X
-0.70 Parasite Toxins 100X
-7.77 Peripheral Nervous System 400X
0.70 Pesticide Toxins 8X
-0.71 Pituitary Gland 1X
-12.04 Potassium Iodide-ch 3X
-9.98 Rayon 24X
-26.16 Salicylic Acid 100X
-0.72 Skin 4000X
-9.15 Small Intestine 15X
11.97 Sodium Eethyl Mercuri 4000X
27.83 Sodium Lauryl Sulfate or Sodium Laureth Sulfate 1000X
15.69 Soft Scrub Cleanser 500X
0.72 Spleen 4000X
5.04 Stomach 8X
-2.10 Structural Reactions 1X
13.66 Sunflower Oil 700X
13.48 Superheated Vegetable Fat 1000X
-13.00 Sweet & Low 100X
-16.27 TV 5X
13.64 Taenia Solium 15X
2.16 Thyroid 24X
11.61 Trichloroethylene 8X
15.61 Trihalomethanes 30X
10.80 Uranium 15X
0.71 Urinary Bladder 7X
2.84 Uterus 5X
11.52 Vitamin B5 400X
-3.50 Vitamins and Minerals Collection 4000X
-15.34 White Wine 1X
-12.05 Zinc Oxide 4000X
15.10 Zirconium 40X

Balancer Results

	Baseline (53)	Product A (29)	Product B (20)	Product C (18)	Product D (14)	Product E (13)
Salicylic Acid	-26.16	4.30	-3.79	5.47	-11.86	-3x57
Chlordane	-19.93	4.99	4.97	-10.23	12.22	-16.60
Central Nervous System	-35.35	5.29	13.53	-12.88	-8.46	11.19
E. Coli	15.46	3.64	-6.94	15.59	6.72	10.65
Mycoplasma Pneumoniae	36.88	-10.35	5.48	-6.64	-5.20	9.66
Agaricus muscarius -mf	10.17	20.35	8.85	-6.93	-4.42	-7.97
Electronic Wireless Toxins	-8.26	-8.22	-11.50	-15.38	-3.34	7.26
Acetone	15.08	-7.97	3.91	-14.09	-4.42	6.30
Rayon	-9.96	-3.22	15.62	7.89	-20.34	5.19
Uranium	10.80	-7.11	4.26	-24.72	10.75	-4.99
Trihalomethanes	15.61	-4.44	3.92	11.10	-8.49	4.22
Liver	-7.71	13.51	-4.05	-4.74	4.44	4.13

 ZYTO™

ZYTO decision support technology does not identify, diagnose, or treat any disease or medical condition and is not a substitute for professional medical advice. Consult with your primary care physician before modifying your lifestyle, diet, or supplement regimen.
- 8/14/2017

Dr. Harold Steinberg, D.C.

Metaldehyde	-11.53	5.89	14.12	-10.25	14.52	-3.99
Potassium Iodide-ch	-12.04	-13.02	3.80	8.88	10.23
Sweet & Low	-13.00	3.81	15.09	32.13
Lysol Pine Action	-39.06	52.20	-4.14	19.80
Lead	10.32	4.53	3.98	-8.11
Dexarcmycotina	-12.46	-5.41	7.52	4.81
2% Milk	10.71	4.58	10.83
Mercury	10.81	3.06	-4.84
Candida stonan	17.88	-44.00
Stomach	5.04	19.44
Alarm Clock	-19.47	-16.20
Cadmium	19.94	-14.61
Trichloroethylene	11.81	-13.05
Superheated Vegetable Fat	13.48	9.34
Lung	5.89	7.57
TV	-19.27	-5.14
Taenia Solium	12.84	-3.50
Sodium Lauryl Sulfate or Sodium Laureth Sulfate	27.83
Soft Scrub Cleanser	19.69
White Wine	-15.34
Zirconium	15.10
Sunflower Oil	13.66
Green Tea	-13.23
BHA & BHT	-13.21
Omega-3 (Linolenic Acid)	-12.19
Zinc Oxide	-12.05
Sodium Ethyl Mercuri	11.97
Vitamin B5	11.52
Adrenal Glands	-10.70
Small Intestine	-9.15
Chemical Toxins	-8.14
Peripheral Nervous System	-7.77
Joints/Connective Tissue	6.49
Hypothalamus Gland	5.80
Arteries/Veins	5.17
Gallbladder	-5.00
Essential Fatty Acids Collection	-4.78
Negative Emotions	4.20
Environmental Toxins	-4.06
Vitamins and Minerals Collection	-3.50
Food Reactions Collection	-3.44

Case Study 5: Bacteria, Lead, Pollen, Environmental, Candida, Lyme Toxins

Mr. J is a 67-year-old nurse who was complaining about low back, knee, ankle and foot pain. The Detox Focus Bio Survey results shows joint and tissue stress, digestive issues with large intestine stress and stressed organ problems with skin and liver.

The list of stressors at the bottom of that chart shows bacteria, lead, pollen and grasses, environmental, candida and Lyme at levels exceeding his base line of 3.52. As a child he was bitten by ticks a few times and does remember a bull's eye mark on his right leg. He never associated tick bites with his health conditions.

The specific remedy recommended for him was a Lyme nosode and a vegetarian digestive enzyme. The first remedy brought 34 stressors down to 23 and the digestive enzyme brought it down to 11. We did not attempt to balance all stressors but just emphasized the Lyme and digestive enzymes.

Dr. Harold Steinberg, D.C.

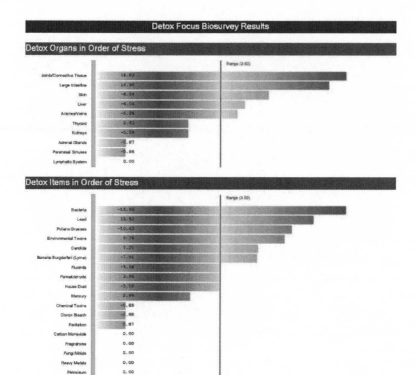

Detox Focus Biosurvey Results

Detox Organs in Order of Stress

Range (3.52)

Joints/Connective Tissue	16.82
Large Intestine	14.96
Skin	-6.54
Liver	-6.04
Arteries/Veins	-5.24
Thyroid	2.61
Kidneys	-3.55
Adrenal Glands	-0.87
Paranasal Sinuses	-0.86
Lymphatic System	0.00

Detox Items in Order of Stress

Range (3.52)

Bacteria	-15.65
Lead	11.62
Pollens Grasses	-10.43
Environmental Toxins	9.79
Candida	7.25
Borrelia Burgdorferi (Lyme)	-7.01
Fluorids	-3.56
Formaldehyde	3.56
House Dust	-3.56
Mercury	2.49
Chemical Toxins	-0.89
Clorox Bleach	-0.86
Radiation	0.87
Carbon Monoxide	0.00
Fragrances	0.00
Fungi/Molds	0.00
Heavy Metals	0.00
Petroleum	0.00
Virus	0.00

Toxic Overload

Detox Balancers

Product A	1 Tablet 1 times per day
Product B	1 Tablespoon 1 times per day
Product C	1 Capsule 3 times per day
Product D	1 Tablespoon 1 times per day
Product E	3 Tablets 1 times per day

Foods to Avoid

We tested 100 foods. These are the top foods you reacted to. The higher the number, the more stressing the food. Reaction numbers greater than 20 are higher reactive foods.

If the number is negative this food potentially makes you more tired. If the number is a high positive it can cause you to over-react, or be more stressed if eaten too often.

Look for food groups (dairy, grains, additives, sugars) or related foods (acid forming foods) in the list. Watch your reaction to the foods listed when you eat them again.

-24.92 **White Wine**

21.17 **Shrimp**

16.89 **Superheated Vegetable Fat**

-16.30 **Fructose**

-16.09 **2% Milk**

15.20 **Corn**

-14.50 **Orange (Fruit)**

-13.11 **White Wheat Flour**

-12.82 **Salt**

12.47 **Egg White**

11.46 **Whole Wheat**

-11.11 **Tuna Fish**

10.90 **Barley**

10.67 **Soy Bean**

10.43 **FD&C Blue No.2**

10.04 **Sunflower Oil**

9.94 **Bakers Yeast**

8.84 **Grape (Red & Green)**

8.84 **Sodium Nitrate**

8.11 **Canola Oil**

133

Balancer Results Comparison

	Baseline (84)	Product A (23)	Product B (11)	Product C (9)	Product D (5)	Product E (4)
White Wine	-34.92	6.19	-6.23	-15.50	3.73	25.41
Sodium Nitrate	8.84	10.25	3.66	14.03	12.26	16.25
House Dust	-3.56	20.35	3.62	-6.48	-3.61	3.74
Skin	-8.54	7.50	-4.56	11.86	-14.96	3.73
Joints/Connective Tissue	16.32	12.55	5.65	5.11	4.90	
Large Intestine	14.96	3.71	-3.62	20.83		
Arteries/Veins	-5.26	-5.20	-22.78	6.51		
Corn	16.20	-34.07	-19.08	5.01		
Liver	-6.04	-6.05	3.67	-3.55		
Superheated Vegetable Fat	16.59	16.21	16.20			
Bacteria	-16.65	7.42	6.94			
2% Milk	-16.09	-23.62				
White Wheat Flour	-13.11	20.39				
Fructose	-16.30	-20.16				
Barley	10.90	-16.79				
Grape (Red & Green)	8.84	-12.72				
Fluoride	-3.56	-12.29				
Salt	-12.92	10.97				
Egg White	11.47	10.73				
Formaldehyde	3.56	6.38				
Candida	7.21	6.23				
Orange (Fruit)	-14.50	-4.07				
Environmental Toxins	9.76	3.79				
Shrimp	21.17					
Lead	12.52					
Whole Wheat	11.46					
Tuna Fish	-11.11					
Soy Bean	10.57					
FD&C Blue No.2	10.43					
Pollens/Grasses	-10.43					
Sunflower Oil	10.04					
Bakers Yeast	6.94					
Canola Oil	8.11					
Borrelia Burgdorferi (Lyme)	-7.01					

Case Study 6: Glyphosate, Arsenic Toxins

Mrs. G, age 38, is a teacher with major respiratory and kidney issues. Since moving to a larger city, she has experienced problems with her energy levels, has been susceptible to colds and her allergy levels have increased dramatically.

Running a detailed report was needed to see what her worst stress areas are. Organ Reactions and Areas of Stress is another report generated to show stressors she is experiencing. Her level of acceptable stress is 8.98. Top Items out of balance by categories further defines the areas of stress that are affecting her health. As an example, her environmental toxin glyphosate level is -18.46 which a stress level higher than her acceptable level of 8.98. Glyphosate is a base of Roundup.

Heavy metals show arsenic at level 13.85 which is higher than the 8.98. Arsenic is prevalent in rice and that is an item she eats regularly. The Balancers page address the supplements needed to balance her stressors. We only picked the first two items that covered 42 of the 46 conditions due to monetary issues on her part.

Dr. Harold Steinberg, D.C.

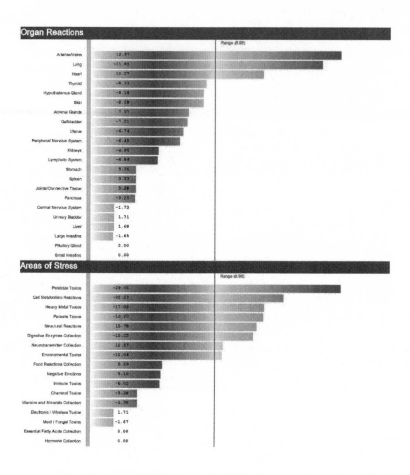

Toxic Overload

Top Items Out of Balance by Category

Cell Metabolism Reactions
-17.66 Protein Metabolism
-17.31 Fat Metabolism
13.61 Methylation
-13.42 Uric Acid-phb
-13.11 Lactic Acid

Digestive Enzymes Collection
12.46 Pepsin

Environmental Toxins
20.80 Feather, Mix
20.65 Fur Mix
-18.46 Glyphosate
-15.55 Pollens Grasses
-13.60 Henna
12.89 Chlorox
11.12 Sawdust, Mixed

Heavy Metal Toxins
-24.61 Platinum
-20.53 Nickel -hm
-19.52 Zirconium
13.95 Arsenic-hm

Parasite Toxins
18.72 Echinococcus Multilo
18.53 Giardia Lamblia
-11.77 Clonorchis Sinensis
10.66 Taenia Saginata

Pesticide Toxins
27.81 Dichloropropene
-20.28 DCPA
-19.81 Prowl
19.48 2,4-D
-18.46 Glyphosate
15.93 Carbofuran
-15.22 Diazinon
14.86 Propanil
14.30 Coal Tar/ Creosote
-13.85 Heptachlor
-12.35 Creosote
-10.81 Boric Acid

Structural Reactions
-16.35 Muscle, Pectoral Complex
16.06 Nerve, Sciatic
13.99 Cervical Vertebrae

Dr. Harold Steinberg, D.C.

Balancers

76.52	Product A	1 Tablet 3 times per day
42.48	Product B	2 Capsules 3 times per day
38.91	Product C	1 Capsule 3 times per day
37.18	Product D	2 Capsules 1 times per day
36.67	Product E	2 Tablets 3 times per day

Potency Results on Stressors

19.48	2,4-D 4000X
-20.23	Cell Metabolism Reactions 4000X
-20.28	DCPA 7X
27.81	Dichloropropene 500X
18.53	Giardia Lamblia 7X
-20.53	Nickel -hm 1000X
-16.92	Parasite Toxins 3X
-29.66	Pesticide Toxins 500X
-24.61	Platinum 4000X
-17.66	Protein Metabolism 400X
-19.52	Zirconium 500X

Balancer Results

	Baseline (46)	Product A (27)	Product B (13)	Product C (4)	Product D (2)	Product E (1)
Environmental Toxins	-10.04	-18.83	-9.12	27.78	28.24	-22.55
Heavy Metal Toxins	-17.05	-14.19	-9.21	-9.21	-11.54	
Nerve, Sciatic	18.05	17.50	11.78	11.70		
Lactic Acid	-13.11	23.91	12.92	-11.26		
Protein Metabolism	-17.66	15.09	23.91			
Taenia Saginata	10.88	38.05	-20.41			
Cervice Vertebrae	13.93	14.35	14.12			
Propanil	14.88	30.52	13.97			
Arsenic-hm	13.85	9.31	13.85			
Creosote	-12.35	-15.21	-13.82			
Pesticide Toxins	-29.66	-14.43	-13.37			
Papain	12.48	-11.17	9.62			
Uric Acid-crb	-13.42	18.30	9.46			
Clonorchis Sinensis	-11.27	-35.92				
Fat Metabolism	-17.21	27.19				
Heart	10.27	25.30				
2,4-D	19.48	-23.53				
Henna	-13.80	19.23				
Echinococcus Mi-sto	15.72	-9.62				
Boric Acid	-10.81	-17.69				
Digestive Enzymes Collection	15.23	17.30				
Arteries/Veins	12.37	-16.30				
Diazinon	-15.22	12.22				
Carbofuran	15.83	11.98				
Heptachlor	-13.55	11.76				

Toxic Overload

Fur Mix	20.65	9.67
Neurotransmitter Collection	10.27	-9.93
Dichloropropene	27.81	
Platinum	24.51	
Feather Mix	20.60	
Nickel-Krin	-20.53	
DCPA	-20.29	
Cell Metabolism Reactions	-20.22	
Prowl	-19.81	
Zirconium	-19.52	
Giardia Lamblia	18.53	
Glyphosate	-18.40	
Parasite Toxins	16.82	
Muscle: Pectoral Complex	-16.34	
Structural Reactions	15.78	
Pollens Grasses	-15.50	
Coal Tar/ Creosote	14.30	
Methylation	13.51	
Clitabox	12.89	
Lung	-11.85	
Sawdust, Mixed	11.12	

Case Study 7: Viral and Bacterial Infections and Immune System

Mrs. G is 47-year-old chemistry scientist, working in high tech areas of a national lab. She has had many issues with viruses and bacterial infections over the past 5 years. Her detox organ stress level is 4.67.

She feels her immune system may be compromised with the environment she is exposed to daily. The page 1 of stressors list radiation, mercury, petroleum and heavy metals as detoxification issues. The organs affected are her large intestines and her joints.

We looked at food sensitivity issues but didn't feel they were of major substance. She did take the recommendation of a rotation diet for the top food items to see if benefits would occur. Page 3 shows the first product balanced 28 stressed items down to 10. The recommended product was a homeopathic mercury detox together with other heavy metals. The next product was 10 items down to 3 with a flower remedy used to balance radiation, Yarrow.

Toxic Overload

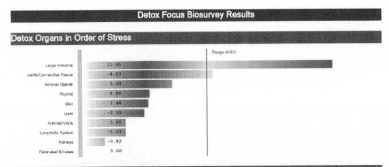

Detox Focus Biosurvey Results

Detox Organs in Order of Stress

Range (4.67)

Organ	Value
Large Intestine	11.45
Joints/Connective Tissue	-4.93
Adrenal Glands	3.14
Thymid	2.50
Skin	2.48
Liver	-2.33
Arteries-Veins	1.66
Lymphatic System	-1.63
Kidneys	-0.82
Paranasal Sinuses	0.00

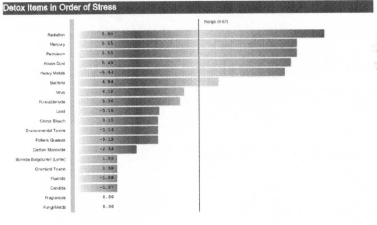

Detox Items in Order of Stress

Range (4.67)

Item	Value
Radiation	5.80
Mercury	5.55
Petroleum	5.55
House Dust	5.49
Heavy Metals	-5.44
Bacteria	4.84
Virus	4.18
Formaldehyde	3.96
Lead	-3.16
Clorox Bleach	3.15
Environmental Toxins	-3.14
Pollens Grasses	-3.13
Carbon Monoxide	-2.14
Borrelia Burgdorferi (Lyme)	1.58
Chemical Toxins	2.58
Fluoride	-1.88
Candida	-1.57
Fragrances	0.00
Fungi/Molds	0.00

Dr. Harold Steinberg, D.C.

Detox Balancers

Product A	1 Tablet 3 times per day
Product B	1 Tablet 3 times per day
Product C	1 Capsule 3 times per day
Product D	2 Capsules 3 times per day
Product E	1 Tablet 1 times per day

Foods to Avoid

We tested 100 foods. These are the top foods you reacted to. The higher the number, the more stressing the food. Reaction numbers greater than 20 are higher reactive foods.

If the number is negative this food potentially makes you more tired. If the number is a high positive it can cause you to over-react, or be more stressed if eaten too often.

Look for food groups (dairy, grains, additives, sugars) or related foods (acid forming foods) in the list. Watch your reaction to the foods listed when you eat them again.

22.54	**Salt**
-13.46	**Canola Oil**
-13.10	**Rye**
12.44	**Chocolate**
11.56	**Egg White**
-11.56	**Gluten**
11.26	**Banana**
10.60	**Mayonnaise**
-10.04	**BHA & BHT**
9.76	**Navy Bean (White)**
-9.74	**White Wheat Flour**
-9.49	**Chicken Meat**
-9.17	**Almond**
9.00	**Yogurt**
-8.66	**Oat**
8.58	**Black Tea**
-8.05	**Grape (Red & Green)**
8.05	**Tomato**
8.03	**MSG**
8.00	**Strawberry**

Toxic Overload

Balancer Results Comparison

	Baseline (28)	Product A (10)	Product B (3)	Product C (2)	Product D (1)	Product E (0)
Navy Bean (White)	9.79	7.82	-4.81	9.31	5.67	
Canola Oil	-13.46	20.48	5.51	8.56		
Salt	22.64	-18.38	-5.99			
Chocolate	12.44	10.20				
Mayonnaise	13.68	-8.78				
Chicken Meat	-9.49	8.56				
MSG	8.03	-8.31				
Bacteria	4.84	7.09				
Petroleum	9.55	6.02				
Yogurt	9.09	5.51				
Rye	13.10					
Egg White	11.56					
Gluten	-11.58					
Large Intestine	11.45					
Banana	11.26					
BHA & BHT	10.04					
White Wheat Flour	9.74					
Almond	-9.17					
Owl	-8.86					
Black Tea	8.58					
Grape (Red & Green)	-8.55					
Tomato	8.05					
Strawberry	8.00					
Radiation	5.80					
Mercury	5.55					
House Dust	5.49					
Heavy Metals	-5.44					
Joints/Connective Tissue	-4.93					

Case Study 8: Organs, Vertebra, including Pollutants, Chemicals, Heavy Metals, Bacteria, Viral, Fungal and Parasite Toxins.

75-year-old, Mr. R, wanted a comprehensive metabolism scan done to see his health level and if there were any stresses he needed to be aware of. The patient did not share much information about his health condition. He was interested in seeing what the reports would show and then talk about his health condition. The following report was produced. Mr. R's stress score was 10.12. In looking at areas that stress his body, we need to look at items greater than 10.12 either as a positive or negative number in the reports. The reason a number can be negative or positive is based on the severity of its stress level. The negative numbers are more stress than its equivalent positive number. I normally make the number an absolute number, so they are all positive numbers.

The Comprehensive Metabolism Report shows stress condition of his skin, at -22.86, joints/connective tissues at 22.41, pancreas at -17.71 heart at -16.71 and large intestine at 15.86. He has had skin dermatitis for years with removal of many skin tags plus removal of "cancer" like skin moles. He does have knee arthritic problems and is scheduled for one full knee replacement. He does have high blood pressure and is on blood pressures medicines and heart drugs to reduce heart rate. The reason the large intestine is showing up, he thinks, is because he has difficulty moving his bowels every day. He reviewed the report and had a positive opinion of the results.

On the spinal stresses at the bottom of the page there is a chart of the stressed vertebra. C2 affects the blood flow to the head and hearing and the tongue and sinuses, L3 the bladder, prostate, and genitals, Thoracic 2 affects the heart and valves of the heart and the lungs, Thoracic 4 nerves go to the gallbladder and heart and lungs, Thoracic 7 innervates the pancreas, esophagus and duodenum.

The next chart shows the top ten internal stressors including hormones, neurotransmitters with nutritional imbalances. The homeopathic balancers are shown with the stressors.

Also listed are the external stress items including pollutants, chemicals, heavy metals, bacteria, viral, fungal and parasites. His body may have these stressors or is just sensitive to them. The homeopathic balances are presented.

This followed by positive statements needed to change his thoughts and his life. These mantras are needed to be repeated to change negative feelings that affect his health and mental attitude to his health.

The Balancer Results Comparison lists all the stressors on the left. The baseline column lists the numeric stress number, greater than 10.12, followed by the five nutritional supplements used to balance all but one stress item. It shows the first nutritional supplement will balance 60 of the 89 items. The second will balance 25 of the remaining 29. The third will balance 3 of the last 4 items leaving 1 item not balanced.

Dr. Harold Steinberg, D.C.

This innovative ZYTO decision support technology helps to discover information specific to your body's unique needs. We call this your biological preference. Using biocommunication, we are able to gather a vast amount of data about your body. This scan is a stimulus-response exchange between the software and your body. The responses generated by your body's energetic system provide valuable information at a level of which you are most likely not conscious.

Using this biocommunication technology you can discover specific, individualized information that will help design a personalized health and nutrition program specific to your body's needs. This individualized scan provides insights and information that can make a significant health difference.

Your Highest Organ Markers

This graph lists the top 5 most potentially stressed organ biomarkers. The higher the value the better probability that the organ many be in need of support. This technology does not diagnose or treat disease or illness, but gives you information on items that may be causing you excess stress.

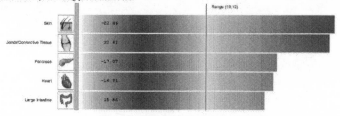

Spinal Stressors

Another factor in making sure your system is in balance is to make sure your vertebrae in your spine are aligned well. The next graph shows you the top 5 vertebrae that can use extra care right now.

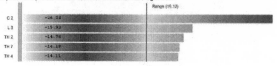

ZYTO decision-support technology does not identify, diagnose, or treat any disease or medical condition and is not a substitute for professional medical advice. Consult with your primary care physician before modifying your lifestyle, diet, or supplement regimen.
- 3/22/2017

Toxic Overload

Our metabolism is controlled by internal and external factors. Internal factors such as hormones, neurotransmitters, along with nutritional imbalances can cause more stress on our system. This list shows you the top 10 metabolism factors to consider.

-56.31 **Epinephrine 4000X**
-42.89 **Aldosterone -hor 7X**
41.08 **Dopamine 30X**
32.03 **Cortisol -h 5X**
26.40 **Serotonin 30X**
22.15 **Norepinephrine 30X**
-21.39 **Iodine 4000X**
18.69 **Cholesterol 4000X**
17.19 **Biotin-vi 400X**
16.12 **Glucagon -h 10X**

Daily we are exposed to many external stress items like environmental pollutants, chemicals, heavy metals, bacteria, viral, fungal, and /or parasites. This list shows the top 10 external stress items for you. This does not mean you have these toxins in your system, just that your body overreacts to these stressors currently.

77.16 **Pollens Trees and Shrubs 3X**
69.88 **Penicillin 10X**
-67.15 **Pollens Flowers 3X**
58.67 **Trichloroethylene 30X**
56.35 **Pneumococcal Pneumonia 24X**
-56.17 **Cytomegalovirus Nos. 10X**
-55.00 **Leishmania Tropica 30X**
43.46 **Johnson grass smut 1000X**
38.77 **Pollens Grasses 100X**
-38.68 **Toxocara Cati 3X**

Your thoughts create your feelings,
Your feelings create your actions,
Your actions create your results.

Change your thoughts - Change your life!

The following 3 statements resonant with your system currently. Repeat each statement a number of times out loud and notice the feelings that come up. Do they make you feel better? Use the statements that feel best to you as affirmations to receive what you desire.

I am safe and calm during the healing process
My body is healed, restored and filled with energy
I nurture my physical body in healthy and loving ways

 ZYTO

ZYTO decision support technology does not identify, diagnose, or treat any disease or medical condition and is not a substitute for professional medical advice. Consult with your primary care physician before modifying your lifestyle, diet, or supplement regimen.
- 3/22/2017

Page 2 of 7

Dr. Harold Steinberg, D.C.

One goal of metabolism balancing is to reduce inflammation caused by food reactions. Common foods that often cause inflammation are all types of sugar including fructose and fruit juice, artificial sweeteners, processed soy, gluten-based grains, genetically-modified corn, and dairy. We do not evaluate these potentially inflammatory foods as a preference for you.

We evaluated four categories of foods (Fruits, Vegetables, Proteins, and Other) to find out what you prefer in each category. The best or most preferred foods are at the top of the list, and the least preferred foods are at the bottom of the list. It is recommended to avoid the bottom 5 foods on each list.

Fruits

Banana
Apple
Grape (Red & Green)
Nectarine
Cantaloupe
Lime
Plum
Papaya
Mango
Raspberry
Cherry
Blueberry
Grapefruit
Lemon
Pineapple
Strawberry
Pear
Watermelon
Oranges
Honeydew Melon
Peach

Vegetables

Beet
Zucchini
Brussel Sprouts
Broccoli
Bean Sprouts
Pepper, Bell
Kale
Lettuce, Leaf
Carrot
Cucumber
String Bean (Green)
Onion
Spinach
Cabbage
Pea, Green
Tomato
Collard Greens
Lettuce, Romaine
Cauliflower
Asparagus

Celery

Proteins

Shrimp
Lobster
Beef
Perch
Halibut
Egg, Whole
Turkey, Dark Meat
Veal
Whitefish
Tilapia
Albacore
Turkey, White Meat
Codfish
Tuna Fish
Chicken, White Meat
Mutton (Lamb)
Salmon
Chicken, Dark Meat

Other Foods

Sunflower Seed
Psyllium Seed
Almond
Coconut Oil
Olive Oil
Coconut
Garbanzo Bean (Chickpeas)
Pinto Bean
Flax Seed
Cashew Nut
Almond Milk
Walnut, English
Black Bean
Rice, Brown
Avocado
Oat
Navy Bean (White)

Dr. Harold Steinberg, D.C.

Here is a list of supplements or remedies you prefer

Product A
Product B
Product C

Baseline
Biomarkers Out of Range: 89

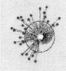

Product A
Biomarkers Brought Into Range: 60
Category:
Usage Directions: 2 1/4 Milliliters 1 times per day

Product B
Additional BioMarkers Brought Into Range: 25
Category:

Product C
Additional BioMarkers Brought Into Range: 3
Category:

ZYTO decision-support technology does not identify, diagnose, or treat any disease or
medical condition and is not a substitute for professional medical advice.
Consult with your primary care physician before modifying your lifestyle, diet, or supplement regimen.
- 3/22/2017

Page 5 of 7

150

Toxic Overload

	Baseline (89)	Product A (29)	Product B (4)	Product C (1)	Product D (1)	Product E (1)
Methanol	23.86	13.18	12.33	-11.24	14.30	22.24
Cytomegalovirus Nos.	-58.17	12.95	-19.70			
11-Deoxycortisol	16.06	-21.89	16.37			
17a-Hydroxypregnenolone	-11.60	-13.89	10.31			
Epinephrine	-56.31	31.43				
Rubella Nos	16.81	-30.06				
Power Lines	-14.57	-28.94				
C 2	-26.04	-23.23				
Rhodotorula Rubra	14.24	21.26				
Toxocara Canis	15.92	-20.95				
Dog Hair	-22.12	-19.08				
iron-hm	-29.17	-17.53				
Penicillin	80.88	17.50				
Johnson grass smut	-43.46	-17.16				
TH 4	-14.11	-16.41				
Ethyl	-16.62	16.06				
Bermuda Grass Smut	11.58	15.00				
E. Coli	-34.61	-14.40				
Klebsiella	-14.70	-13.11				
Rayon	12.89	-12.89				
Aldosterone Fol	42.99	-2.65				
Glyphosate	-19.34	12.53				
Poison Weeds	22.76	11.41				
Cholecystokinin	-14.35	11.24				
Agaricus muscarius -mf	33.47	-10.98				
Iodine	-21.39	-10.96				
Brain	-47.11	13.76				
Petroleum	15.63	10.89				
Pneumococcal Pneumonia	55.35	-10.55				
Pollens Trees and Shrubs	77.18					
Pollens Flowers	-67.15					
Trichloroethylene	55.67					
Leishmania Tropica	-56.06					
Dopamine	41.08					
Pollens Grasses	33.77					
Toxocara Cati	36.86					
Nail Fungus	-36.07					
Entamoeba Gingivalis	-32.25					
Cortisol -f	32.03					
Paragonimus Westermani	31.43					
Enterovirus	28.64					
Cigarette Smoke	28.60					
Enterobius Verm (OX)	28.64					
Otitis Media Nos.	-27.82					
Mononucleosis, Infectious	-26.74					
Benfotin	26.40					
Tuberculinum	-26.75					
Pertussis (Bordetela)	25.08					
DMDM Hydantoin & Urea (Imidazolidinyl)	-24.96					
Skin	22.86					

3/22/2017

151

Dr. Harold Steinberg, D.C.

Joints/Connective Tissue	22.41					
Norepinephrine	22.15					
Epstein Barr Virus	21.28					
Paint Thinner	-20.98					
Mucor racemosus	-19.78					
Cell Phone	-19.04					
Toxoplasma Gondii Nos	-18.38					
Cholesterol	18.69					
Aluminum	17.08					
Potassium Iodide ch	-17.80					
Biotin-x	17.19					
Pancreas	-17.07					
Uranium	16.79					
Clostridium Diffici	16.74					
Heart	-16.71					
Glucagon -h	16.12					
L 5	-15.93					
Large Intestine	15.86					
Alcohol ch	15.78					
Lactic Acid	15.49					
17a-Hydroxyprogesterone	-15.47					
Low Lox	15.44					
Adrenalin	15.23					
TH 2	-14.76					
Lead	-14.75					
Dientamoeba Fragilis	-14.59					
TH 7	14.19					
Silver	14.09					
Cerium	-13.97					
Pregnenolone	13.38					
Lung Fungus	13.26					
Gold	-12.79					
Botulismus	12.05					
Arsenic	11.68					
Asbestos	-11.53					
Copper	11.52					
Corynebacterium Anaerobius	-11.40					
T4 - Thyroxine	-11.25					
Acetylcholine Chloride	10.48					

Case Study 9: Bacteria, Environmental, Adrenals, Aspartame Toxins

Mr. J, an 82-year-old is retired with memory issues, muscle pains and knee and hip joint pain. His medical doctors say his health is good and his blood tests are in normal range.

We sat for a few minutes and talked about his prescription medicines and over the counter drugs he is taking. He is on a statin drug and is taking 4 Advil a day. His blood lab tests looked good. His cholesterol was at 140 and his CRP was in normal range. His weight is at a constant level for years and he is not fat. He said his diet is good and does not drink alcohol, but he does drink diet sodas and diet tea.

We looked at different detox groups and found a high bacteria stress level of -71.08 and environmental stress level of -70.97. His stress level was 15.47. His adrenals and arteries/veins had stress of -40.57 and 38.11 respectively. Two homeopathic products were used to create a balanced state. The 33 items balanced to 3.

But an important item showed on page 2 of the report. Aspartame was at a level of high stress at 244.68. That was the issue with muscle and joint pain. We agreed to get off aspartame. Within three weeks his pains were gone.

The other issue was a cholesterol level of 140. This is quite low. With conversations with his MD we removed the statin over a few weeks and with a level of 180 his memory is quite normal.

Dr. Harold Steinberg, D.C.

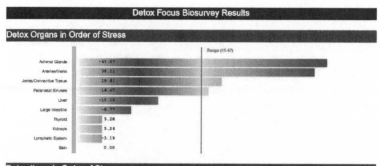

Detox Focus Biosurvey Results

Detox Organs in Order of Stress

Range (15.47)

Organ	Value
Adrenal Glands	-48.57
Arteries/Veins	38.11
Joints/Connective Tissue	19.41
Paranasal Sinuses	18.47
Liver	-18.15
Large Intestine	-6.77
Thyroid	3.26
Kidneys	3.24
Lymphatic System	-3.19
Skin	0.00

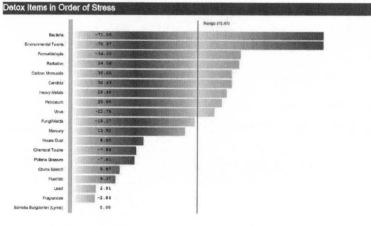

Detox Items in Order of Stress

Range (15.47)

Item	Value
Bacteria	-71.04
Environmental Toxins	-76.97
Formaldehyde	-34.23
Radiation	34.04
Carbon Monoxide	30.68
Candida	30.43
Heavy Metals	28.49
Petroleum	25.89
Virus	-22.76
Fungi/Molds	-16.27
Mercury	13.92
House Dust	8.99
Chemical Toxins	-7.89
Pollens/Grasses	-7.61
Clorox Bleach	5.97
Fluoride	5.27
Lead	2.91
Fragrances	-2.84
Borrelia Burgdorferi (Lyme)	0.00

154

Toxic Overload

Detox Balancers

Product A	2 Tablets 4 times per day
Product B	3 Drops 3 times per day
Product C	3 Drops 3 times per day

Foods to Avoid

We tested 100 foods. These are the top foods you reacted to. The higher the number, the more stressing the food. Reaction numbers greater than 20 are higher reactive foods.

If the number is negative this food potentially makes you more tired. If the number is a high positive it can cause you to over-react, or be more stressed if eaten too often.

Look for food groups (dairy, grains, additives, sugars) or related foods (acid forming foods) in the list. Watch your reaction to the foods listed when you eat them again.

244.68	Aspartame
-99.00	Coffee
-86.27	Apple
62.86	Cheese, Swiss
55.00	Sugar, Maple
53.99	Eggplant
52.68	Chicken Meat
46.93	Egg, White
-45.88	Soy Bean
41.78	Chocolate
38.56	Tea, Green
-37.89	Banana
-36.31	Corn
34.20	Rice, White
34.17	Wine, Red
-33.56	Cheese, American
33.05	Fructose
-31.81	Cheese, Cheddar
31.27	Canola Oil
30.80	Sodium Nitrate

Dr. Harold Steinberg, D.C.

Balancer Results Comparison

	Baseline (33)	Product A (11)	Product B (3)	Product C (0)
Sugar, Maple	55.00	44.81	37.08	
Chocolate	41.78	47.57	26.83	
Egg, White	46.93	15.71	17.25	
Aspartame	244.68	148.67		
Apple	-86.27	69.76		
Banana	-37.89	40.89		
Candida	30.43	30.43		
Tea, Green	38.56	-24.82		
Coffee	-82.00	19.74		
Eggplant	53.99	18.33		
Chrom, Bures	52.66	19.17		
Bacteria	-71.08			
Environmental Toxins	-70.97			
Chicken Meat	52.68			
Soy Bean	-46.88			
Adrenal Glands	40.57			
Arteries/Veins	38.11			
Corn	-36.31			
Formaldehyde	-34.25			
Rice, White	34.20			
Wine, Red	34.17			
Radiation	34.06			
Cheese, American	-33.90			
Fructose	-33.05			
Cheese, Cheddar	31.81			
Canola Oil	31.27			
Sodium Nitrate	30.80			
Carbon Monoxide	30.65			
Heavy Metals	28.49			
Petroleum	25.88			
Virus	22.78			
Joints/Connective Tissue	19.41			
Paranisal Sinuses	18.67			

test male - 3/17/2017

156

Chapter 13 - Foods that are good for you

With the hundreds, if not thousands, of diet books and diet plans you are overwhelmed with all the choices, suggestions and comments from your health care provider, friends, relatives and co-workers. Everyone has a plan for you. Remember that we are all individuals with our own genetic profile. With our own small and large intestinal microbes that make us individuals. We don't eat the same foods as others do. We have different responses to the foods our friends and spouses eat. We are individuals.

My recommendations for foods to eat is based on the lists presented by Dr. Peter D'Adamo in his book *"Diet for Your Blood Type"*. And even then, I tell patients to be aware of food reactions if they can and eliminate foods that cause stomach discomfort, gas, belching or especially heartburn. When the food is being attacked by our immune system we are normally not in peak health. We want our immune system to fight bad guys, the bacteria, viruses, molds and parasites.

Recently the biofeedback system released a food choice program to allow the patient to pick a "diet" type and test the best foods for them to eat plus the top foods to avoid. I have used this program with any diet a patient wants to try. I also use it with Dr. D'Adamo's recommendations.

When the correct foods are eaten patients have lost weight, reduced diabetes type 2, reduced their A1C levels, reduced the blood SED rate number, reduced cholesterol levels and are feeling more energetic with less "arthritic" problems.

In addition to the patient's choices of diet or menu items, there is a section of the biofeedback that will allow the system to recommend foods that are good for you or even of more interest may be the foods to avoid. What one does not want is to have your immune system "fight" foods instead of disease issues.

The following illustrations, "Dairy-Free" and "Paleo" are included to visualize the types of food plans that can be evaluated for each individual.

Dr. Harold Steinberg, D.C.

Food plays a critical role in your overall wellness. While the phrase, "An apple a day keeps the doctor away" is good advice for most, a diet that is optimal for one individual likely won't be optimal for another. This concept is known as bio-individuality.

The Food for Wellness scan addresses your bio-individuality by gathering and displaying readings of food items for which your body showed a biological coherence, or preference, as well as items that your body had an incoherent response to.

Please note that this biosurvey does not identify allergies. Be sure to take any known allergies into consideration when referring to this report to help you make wellness decisions about your diet.

Diet Filters Selected

This report will show only those items that fit into the following selected diet categories, if any:

Dairy-Free

ITEM RESPONSES: POSITIVE dR VALUES BY CATEGORY

Below is a list of your most biologically coherent, or preferred, items separated by food category. These can be incorporated into your diet along with other recommendations made by your practitioner.

Beans & Legumes

Beans & Legumes include any fruit or seed of leguminous plants used for food, which includes beans and peas. According to the USDA, beans and peas fit under both the Vegetable Group and the Protein Group (1). Beans and legumes have high mineral and fiber content without the saturated fat found in some animal proteins. (2)

Pinto Bean 14.54	Navy Bean (White) 11.27	Jicama 9.97
Fava Bean 8.39	Black Bean 6.75	Broad Bean 5.55
Haricot Bean 4.25	Beans Mung 3.68	Tamarind Bean 2.65
Blackeyed Pea 1.85	Cannellini Bean (White) 1.22	Butter Bean 0.00
Edamame 0.06		

Beverages

Beverages that are considered healthy include water, tea, juice, and wine. Water is especially critical for hydration and helps the body eliminate toxic substances (3). Tea originated in China and has been used for medicinal purposes for thousands of years. Drinking wine in moderation has been linked to a healthier heart, stronger bones, and a sharper mind. (4)

Cranberry Juice 12.49	Kombucha 9.82	Spearmint Tea 9.99
Peppermint Tea 8.22	Raspberry Leaf Tea 7.27	Dandelion Tea 7.13
Rosehip Tea 6.34	Mint Tea 4.52	Black Tea 3.53
Purah Tea 2.74	Burdock Tea 2.89	Thyme Tea 2.89
Water 1.83	Alkaline Water 0.89	Coffee 0.00
Red Wine 0.00	White Tea 0.00	

Dairy & Eggs

Dairy includes milk, cheese, butter, and yogurt. It is a good source of calcium, vitamin D, and potassium. Consuming too much dairy, however, has been linked to certain health issues. Eggs consist of a yolk and egg white. As a whole, they are high in protein but not high in fat or calories. (5)

Egg White 17.34	Egg, Whole 0.90

Fats & Oils

Fats & Oils that are considered healthy include certain nut and seed oils, butter, avocado oil, and cod liver oil. The body needs essential fats such as these for energy, cell growth support, hormone production, and nutrient absorption. (6)

Grapeseed Oil 3.58	Sesame Oil 3.56	Avocado Oil 2.87
Walnut Oil 0.88	Coconut Oil 0.00	Macadamia Oil 0.00
Tallow (Beef/Mutton) 0.00		

Fish & Seafood

Fish & Seafood is rich in vitamins, minerals, and protein. It is high in omega-3 fatty acids, which have a number of health benefits. Foods rich in omega-3s such as fish & seafood promote heart, joint, eye, brain, and immune health. (7)

Hickory Nut 0.85	Coconut 0.00	Pecans 0.00
Pine Nut 0.00	Pomegranate Seeds 0.00	Pumpkin Seeds 0.00

Spices & Seasonings

Spices & Seasonings may help protect against certain chronic conditions such as heart disease, cancer, and diabetes, according to WebMD. Certain spices and herbs contain antioxidants, which can curb inflammation in the body. Studies also show that they help with weight control. (13)

Pepper 16.03	Baharat 11.94	Poppy Seed 11.51
Boldo / Boldine 11.39	Fennel 9.93	Monarda 9.59
Black Cumin 9.25	Watercress 9.00	Candlenut 8.77
Juniper 8.86	Jamaican Sorrel 7.99	Chervil 8.16
Epazote 6.13	Black Lime / Loomi 5.80	Lemongrass 5.78
Sage 5.67	Samber Spice Blend 5.63	Savory 5.52
Marjoram 5.36	Grains of Paradise 5.33	Cassia 4.73
Curry 4.47	Sesame 4.84	Bush Tomato / Akudjura 4.01
Lovage 3.90	Vanilla 3.26	Wattleseed 3.22
Szechuan Pepper 3.17	Horseradish 2.57	Angelica 2.55
Quatre Epice 2.43	White Turmeric / Zedoary 2.42	Herbs de Provence 2.37
Cardamom 2.34	Pandan Leaf 2.34	Cumin Seed 1.78
Asafetida 1.68	Kabsa Spice 1.58	Caraway Seed 1.57
Cayenne Pepper 1.57	Snakeweed 1.56	Lemon Verbena 1.56
Paprika 1.54	Chaat Masala 1.54	Clove 1.52
Fenugreek 1.52	Fines Herbs 1.51	Dill 1.46
Aleppo Pepper 0.85	Annatto 0.85	Allspice 0.84
Barberry 0.84	Pickling Spice Recipe 0.81	Calamus aromaticus 0.80

Millet 4.23	Oat 4.18	Quinoa 3.31
Barley 2.56	Teff 2.44	Corn 0.00
Spelt 0.00		

Meats & Poultry

Meats & Poultry contain a large amount of protein, an essential building block of body tissue and source of fuel for the body. Many meats are also rich in iron, zinc, and selenium as well as vitamin A, B, and D (10). On the downside, eating certain meats can potentially harden blood vessels and negatively impact the colon and brain. (11)

Cow Liver 22.37	Chicken Meat 16.10	Moose 11.49
Buffalo 8.66	Chicken Liver 7.86	Quail 6.66
Mutton (Lamb) 5.69	Elk 5.09	Goose 2.52
Turkey Meat 2.40	Cornish Hen 2.23	Pork 0.82

Miscellaneous Foods

Chocolate 12.27	Kelp 7.83	Rice Vinegar 6.88
Soy Sauce 6.87	Carob 5.02	Red Vinegar 2.80
Horseradish 2.97	Pickles 1.70	Ginger 0.87
Balsamic Vinegar 0.00	Barley Malt 0.00	Kimchi 0.00
Miso 0.00	Pimento 0.00	

Nuts & Seeds

Nuts & Seeds contain heart-healthy fats, fiber, protein, and minerals. They can reduce inflammation, slow digestion to help you feel full for longer, and reduce heart and cancer risk. Different nuts contain differing ratios of healthy fats, so consuming a variety in moderation is recommended. (12)

Hazelnut (Filbert) 12.01	English Walnut 9.62	Chia Seed 8.87
Lychee 8.61	Cashew Nut 6.23	Chestnut 6.21
Caraway Seed 5.40	Pistachio 2.54	Black Walnut 1.60
Cumin Seed 1.78	Flax Seed 0.86	Psyllium Seed 0.86

Dr. Harold Steinberg, D.C.

Tamarind 0.80	Panch Phoron 0.78	Chili Powder 0.77
Mandrasi Masala 0.77	Garam Masala 0.76	Garlic 0.76
Ginger 0.76	Capers 0.00	Chervil 0.00
Lemon Myrtle 0.00	Licorice 0.00	Mint 0.00
Nigella 0.00	Nutmeg 0.00	Ras el Hanout 0.00
Saffron 0.00	Scented Geranium 0.00	Turmeric 0.00

Sugars & Sweeteners

Sugars & Sweeteners that are considered healthy include honey, maca, stevia, and agave. These and other good sweeteners provide many benefits such as lowering blood pressure, improving bone density, and feeding good bacteria in the gut. (14)

Maple Sugar 12.15	Balsamic Glaze 9.03	Cane Sugar 8.91
Brown Rice Syrup 8.06	Stevia 7.46	Molasses 7.23
Maple Syrup 6.39	Maca 4.62	Xylitol 3.25
Sorghum Syrup 0.82	Coconut Sugar 0.00	

Vegetables

Vegetables are an important source of nutrients including fiber, folic acid, vitamin A, vitamin C, and potassium. They can help maintain blood sugar, lower the risk of heart disease, reduce constipation, boost the immune system, and keep the teeth and gums, skin, and eyes healthy. (15)

Watercress 15.01	Brussel Sprouts 13.09	Okra 10.23
Scallions 8.48	White Potato 7.86	Water Chestnut 7.84
Endive 7.37	Parsnip 7.14	Broccoli Sprouts 5.52
Romaine Lettuce 6.35	Red Cabbage 6.30	Potato Starch 6.23
Rappini 4.76	Eggplant 4.10	Escarole 4.00
Beet Greens 3.30	Chinese Cabbage 3.28	Avocado 3.26

Toxic Overload

Portabella Mushroom 3.17	Winter Squash 3.13	Palm Hearts 3.09
Horseradish 2.57	Carrot 2.44	Cauliflower 2.44
Celery 2.44	Parsley 2.35	Cucumber 1.61
Leek 1.59	Sweet Potato 1.55	Bean Sprouts 0.82
Kohlrabi 0.79	Red Potato 0.79	Yam 0.77
Corn 0.00	Asparagus 0.00	Beet Root 0.00
Kale 0.00	Mixed Lettuce 0.00	Radicchio 0.00
Tempeh 0.00	Yellow Squash 0.00	

ITEM RESPONSES: TOP NEGATIVE dR VALUES

The following are the top food items your body showed an incoherent biological response to. These are items you may want to consider limiting or eliminating from your diet under the guidance of your practitioner.

Papaya -193.43	Prickly Pear -189.27	Peach -77.62
Prune -21.67	Lentils -21.12	Goat -20.33
Pineapple -15.17	Licorice Tea -14.93	Lima Bean -14.15
Buckwheat -13.41	Yacon Root -12.80	Loganberry -12.55
Basil -12.31	Peanut -11.89	Mackerel -11.71
Senna Tea -11.60	Milk Thistle Tea -11.58	Great Northern Bean (White) -11.53
Echinacea Tea -11.46	Mandarine Orange -11.28	Pepper - Green Red Orange & Yellow -10.66
Veal -10.50	Elderberry / Elderflower -10.44	Kokum -10.31
Persimmon -9.55	Hot Sauce -9.45	Lemon Balm -9.33
Watermelon -9.27	Tamari -9.22	Spaghetti Squash -9.12

Dr. Harold Steinberg, D.C.

Food plays a critical role in your overall wellness. While the phrase, "An apple a day keeps the doctor away" is good advice for most, a diet that is optimal for one individual likely won't be optimal for another. This concept is known as bio-individuality.

The Food for Wellness scan addresses your bio-individuality by gathering and displaying readings of food items for which your body showed a biological coherence, or preference, as well as items that your body had an incoherent response to.

Please note that this biosurvey does not identify allergies. Be sure to take any known allergies into consideration when referring to this report to help you make wellness decisions about your diet.

Diet Filters Selected

This report will show only those items that fit into the following selected diet categories, if any:

Paleo

ITEM RESPONSES: POSITIVE dR VALUES BY CATEGORY

Below is a list of your most biologically coherent, or preferred, items separated by food category. These can be incorporated into your diet along with other recommendations made by your practitioner.

Beans & Legumes

Beans & Legumes include any fruit or seed of leguminous plants used for food, which includes beans and peas. According to the USDA, beans and peas fit under both the Vegetable Group and the Protein Group (1). Beans and legumes have high mineral and fiber content without the saturated fat found in some animal proteins. (2)

Beverages

Beverages that are considered healthy include water, tea, juice, and wine. Water is especially critical for hydration and helps the body eliminate toxic substances (3). Tea originated in China and has been used for medicinal purposes for thousands of years. Drinking wine in moderation has been linked to a healthier heart, stronger bones, and a sharper mind. (4)

Water	Water and Lemon	Licorice Tea
70.33	37.82	32.69
Rooibos Tea	Oolong Tea	Red Wine
26.77	24.55	18.64
Burdock Tea	Coffee	Hawthorn Tea
18.20	12.94	12.08
Green Tea	St. John's Wort Tea	Pureh Tea
6.37	6.59	5.41

Chamomile Tea 4.73	Passion Flower Tea 3.52	Ginger Tea 3.40
Aloe Vera Juice 2.99	Peppermint Tea 1.80	Mint Tea 1.78
Fenugreek Tea 1.60	Alfalfa Tea 1.53	Echinacea Tea 0.00
Milk Thistle Tea 0.00	Raspberry Leaf Tea 0.00	Spearmint Tea 0.00
Yerba Mate Tea 0.00		

Dairy & Eggs

Dairy includes milk, cheese, butter, and yogurt. It is a good source of calcium, vitamin D, and potassium. Consuming too much dairy, however, has been linked to certain health issues. Eggs consist of a yolk and egg white. As a whole, they are high in protein but not high in fat or calories. (5)

Egg, Whole
8.21

Fats & Oils

Fats & Oils that are considered healthy include certain nut and seed oils, butter, avocado oil, and cod liver oil. The body needs essential fats such as these for energy, cell growth support, hormone production, and nutrient absorption. (6)

Walnut Oil 27.23	Tallow (Beef/Mutton) 17.05	Almond Oil 13.33
Flax Seed Oil 6.67	Pumpkin seed Oil 4.98	Sesame Oil 3.38
Cod Liver Oil 3.27	Avocado Oil 1.64	

Fish & Seafood

Fish & Seafood is rich in vitamins, minerals, and protein. It is high in omega-3 fatty acids, which have a number of health benefits. Foods rich in omega-3s such as fish & seafood promote heart, joint, eye, brain, and immune health. (7)

Anchovy 97.35	Mackerel 19.27	Sea Trout 14.45
Oyster 13.98	Herring 13.54	Catfish 10.82
Tilapia 9.81	Haddock 8.94	Bluegill (Bream) 8.83
Salmon - Alaskan/Sockeye 8.06	Crab - Dungeness 7.10	Trout 6.35

Dr. Harold Steinberg, D.C.

Pacific Cod	Coho Salmon	Calamari or Squid
4.80	3.59	3.56
Sardine	Black Cod (Sablefish)	Mussels
3.15	1.52	1.51
Barramundi	Clam	Halibut
0.00	0.00	0.00

Fruits are a good source of vitamins and simple sugars, which are essential for optimal health. Their high fiber content helps with bowel movements and wards off cholesterol. Fruits also contain antioxidants, which can protect the body from stress and disease. Due to their many beneficial properties, fruits can prevent and delay the effects of aging. (8)

Carob	Lime	Apricot
49.42	39.43	33.64
Watermelon	Fig	Apple
17.37	16.55	13.13
Boysenberry	Tangerine	Peach
12.64	11.93	10.37
Pear	Pineapple	Cranberry
10.20	9.42	8.15
Papaya	Black Currant	Starfruit
8.86	8.59	7.41
Coconut	Orange (Fruit)	Date
7.06	5.85	3.78
Lemon	Prune	Grapefruit
3.44	1.39	0.00
Persimmon	Raspberry	Rhubarb
0.00	0.00	0.00

Grains

Grains include wheat, rice, and corn. They provide an abundance of nutrients including fiber, antioxidants, protein, B vitamins, and trace minerals. Consumption of grains can reduce the risk of heart disease, obesity, and diabetes. Grains can also reduce inflammation. However, grains might not be appropriate for certain people such as those with celiac disease or gluten sensitivity. (9)

Corn
12.86

Meats & Poultry contain a large amount of protein, an essential building block of body tissue and source of fuel for the body. Many meats are also rich in iron, zinc, and selenium as well as vitamin A, B, and D (10). On the downside, eating certain meats can potentially harden blood vessels and negatively impact the colon and brain. (11)

Turkey Meat	Pheasant	Moose
12.85	10.00	9.74

Chicken Meat	Rabbit	Beef
9.13	8.24	6.20
Partridge	Cow Liver	Ostrich
4.87	0.00	0.00

Miscellaneous Foods

Carob	Ginger	Pimento
49.42	25.96	19.29
White Vinegar	Miso	Dulse
13.70	6.62	6.45
Horseradish	Kelp	Hot Sauce
4.80	3.32	1.67
Garlic	Chocolate	Balsamic Vinegar
1.58	1.54	0.00
Rice Vinegar		
0.00		

Nuts & Seeds

Nuts & Seeds contain heart-healthy fats, fiber, protein, and minerals. They can reduce inflammation, slow digestion to help you feel full for longer, and reduce heart and cancer risk. Different nuts contain differing ratios of healthy fats, so consuming a variety in moderation is recommended. (12)

Sunflower Seed	Pumpkin Seeds	Pine Nut
23.18	21.58	16.86
Poppyseed	Flax Seed	Sacha Inchi Seed
11.49	11.32	10.15
Sesame Seed	Coconut	Black Walnut
7.13	7.06	6.57
Pomegranate Seeds	Macadamia	Grape Seeds
5.49	3.24	3.10
Anise Seed	Hickory Nut	Carraway Seed
1.69	1.64	1.49
Almond		
0.00		

Spices & Seasonings

Spices & Seasonings may help protect against certain chronic conditions such as heart disease, cancer, and diabetes, according to WebMD. Certain spices and herbs contain antioxidants, which can curb inflammation in the body. Studies also show that they help with weight control. (13)

Cayenne Pepper	Baharat	Scented Geranium
88.64	87.06	68.15
Szechuan Pepper	Grains of Paradise	Celery Seed
44.20	40.31	36.67
Asafetida	Fines Herbs	Curry
36.36	30.16	27.99

ZYTO decision-support technology does not identify, diagnose, or treat any disease or medical condition and is not a substitute for professional medical advice. Consult with your primary care physician before modifying your lifestyle, diet, or supplement regimen.
– 8/16/2017

Dr. Harold Steinberg, D.C.

Jamaican Sorrel 25.05	Pandan Leaf 23.18	Angelica 22.70
Turmeric 21.19	Garam Masala 20.50	Soapwort 16.97
Savory 15.94	Panch Phoron 15.87	Bush Tomato / Akudjura 14.90
Ras el Hanout 14.09	Sumac 13.71	Kaffir Lime 13.07
Cardamom 12.83	Calamus aromaticus 12.25	Aleppo Pepper 12.13
Watercress 11.92	Sesame 10.79	Dill 10.66
Lemon Verbena 10.55	Chives 10.35	Sassafras 9.64
Herbs de Provence 9.33	Black Lime / Loomi 9.32	Pepper 9.10
Bouquet Garni 8.13	Vanilla 8.09	Hyssop 7.86
Juniper 7.43	Kebsa Spice 7.26	Berbere 7.21
Annatto 7.16	Bay Leaf 7.16	Candlenut 7.13
Caraway Seed 6.76	Basil 6.30	Green Masala 6.20
Mint 6.20	Orris Root 6.09	Elderberry / Elderflower 6.07
Wasabi 6.03	Lemongrass 5.91	Horseradish 4.80
Sage 4.70	Pumpkin Pie Spice 4.63	Poppy Seed 4.52
Barberry 4.13	Borage 4.02	Harissa 3.13
Quatre Epice 3.10	Capers 2.03	Wattleseed 1.95
Anise Seed 1.89	Saffron 1.58	Ginger 1.56
Fennel 1.54	Pickling Spice Recipe 1.53	Mandrasi Masala 1.52
Paprika 1.45	Chili Powder 0.99	Kokum 0.00
Mahlab 0.00	Za'atar 0.00	

Sugars & Sweeteners

Toxic Overload

 Sugars & Sweeteners that are considered healthy include honey, maca, stevia, and agave. These and other good sweeteners provide many benefits such as lowering blood pressure, improving bone density, and feeding good bacteria in the gut. (14)

Honey 24.60	Stevia 23.78	Sucanat 9.19
Yacon Root 8.80		

Vegetables

 Vegetables are an important source of nutrients including fiber, folic acid, vitamin A, vitamin C, and potassium. They can help maintain blood sugar, lower the risk of heart disease, reduce constipation, boost the immune system, and keep the teeth and gums, skin, and eyes healthy. (15)

Caraway 212.92	Arugula 86.65	Asparagus 54.05
Celeriac (Celery Root) 51.67	Parsley 23.97	Carrot 22.06
Scallions 19.32	Kale 19.02	Dandelion Greens 16.15
Spaghetti Squash 14.97	Broccoli 14.90	Winter Squash 14.35
Chicory 14.01	Seaweed 13.16	Corn 12.86
Yellow Squash 12.22	Alfalfa Sprouts 11.83	Green Olive 10.97
Lettuce 10.41	Chives 10.35	Jalapenos 9.28
Swiss Chard 9.01	Sweet Potato 7.51	Red Cabbage 7.17
Cucumber 6.71	Bok Choy 6.24	Okra 5.48
Kohlrabi 5.00	Horseradish 4.80	Romaine Lettuce 4.38
Fennel 4.26	Collard Greens 4.09	Daikon 4.09
Eggplant 3.93	Zucchini 3.12	Garlic 1.58
White Cabbage 1.50	Shiitake Mushroom 1.47	Chinese Cabbage 1.38
Portabella Mushroom 1.37	Rhubarb 0.00	Iceberg Lettuce 0.00
Pepper - Green Red Orange & Yellow 0.00	Shallot 0.00	

ZYTO decision-support technology does not identify, diagnose, or treat any disease or medical condition and is not a substitute for professional medical advice. Consult with your primary care physician before modifying your lifestyle, diet, or supplement regimen.
- 8/16/2017

Page 6 of 8

169

Dr. Harold Steinberg, D.C.

ITEM RESPONSES: TOP NEGATIVE dR VALUES

The following are the top food items your body showed an incoherent biological response to. These are items you may want to consider limiting or eliminating from your diet under the guidance of your practitioner.

Butternut Squash -116.85	Cassia -110.46	Chicory Spice -82.15
Chervil -77.45	Clove -72.17	White Wine -63.04
Chili Pepper -57.25	Brussel Sprouts -55.76	Nectarine -49.54
White Tea -44.49	Cherry -33.92	Honeydew Melon -33.85
Cauliflower -32.81	Broccoli Sprouts -32.07	Coconut Sugar -30.59
Maple Sugar -29.05	Dandelion Tea -28.80	Mango -27.37
Molasses -26.79	Rosemary -24.03	Goat -23.49
Cane Sugar -23.48	Valerian Tea -21.42	Blueberry -21.18
Loganberry -20.47	Leek -19.78	Casaba Melon -19.13
Parsley -18.45	Orange Juice -17.25	Brown Rice Syrup -17.16

Toxic Overload

Bibliography:

1. "The Benefits of Beans and Legumes." American Heart Association. https://recipes.heart.org/Articles/1026/The-Benefits-of-Beans-and-Legumes

2. "Beans and peas are unique foods." Choosemyplate.gov. https://recipes.heart.org/Articles/1026/The-Benefits-of-Beans-and-Legumes

3. "The Importance of Proper Hydration" Heritage Integrative Healthcare. http://heritageihc.com/blog/proper-hydration/

4. "Bottoms Up" WebMD. http://www.webmd.com/diet/features/health-benefits-wine#2

5. "The Pros and Cons of Milk and Dairy." WebMD. http://www.webmd.com/diet/healthy-kitchen-11/dairy-truths?page=1

6. "Dietary Fats." American Heart Association. https://healthyforgood.heart.org/Eat-smart/Articles/Dietary-Fats

7. "Top 10 Health Benefits of Eating Seafood." HealthFitnessRevolution.org http://www.healthfitnessrevolution.com/top-10-health-benefits-eating-seafood/

8. Fruit nutrition facts." Nutrition And You.com http://www.nutrition-and-you.com/fruit-nutrition.html

9. "9 Legitimate Health Benefits of Eating Whole Grains." Authority Nutrition. https://authoritynutrition.com/9-benefits-of-whole-grains/

10. "3 Benefits of Eating Meat" Medical Daily. http://www.medicaldaily.com/3-benefits-eating-meat-234798

11. "10 Reasons to Stop Eating Red Meat" Prevention. http://www.prevention.com/food/healthy-eating-tips/10-reasons-to-stop-eating-red-meat

12. "What Are the Health Benefits of Eating Nuts & Seeds?" Livestrong.com. http://www.livestrong.com/article/411381-what-are-the-health-benefits-of-eating-nuts-seeds/

13. "Spices and Herbs: Their Health Benefits" WebMD. http://www.webmd.com/food-recipes/features/spices-and-herbs-health-benefits#2

14. "4 Natural Sweeteners That Are Good for Your Health." Authority Nutrition. https://authoritynutrition.com/4-healthy-natural-sweeteners/

15. "Why is it important to eat vegetables." ChooseMyPlate.gov. https://www.choosemyplate.gov/vegetables-nutrients-health

Chapter 14 - Summary

The examples shown should bring detail to the types of inquiries that can be made for an individual with health concerns. There are many more conditions that can be evaluated. I wanted to show a few different types of studies and the way the bio-feedback system can help.

When I balance a patient, my philosophy is that fewer products are better than more. The nature of our body is to heal itself from the inside out. The better the diet, the better quality of the supplements, the better the homeopathy frequency levels, the faster and the body can heal.

A follow-up visit with the patient is normally scheduled within a month or so after the initial visit. We take another look at the supplements and the diet and homeopathic remedies needed, if any. The most positive is a change in diet and lifestyle.

For all patients, seeing their stress levels and organ systems, opens much communication. The discussions can go back decades and we then can get a better understanding what is compromising their health.

Normally, small changes are made to a patient's lifestyle or diet that has minimal impact on their daily life but are needed to achieve noticeable results. We look at three to six weeks as a reasonable timeframe to see changes occur.

The system has different ways of looking at stress conditions. Each area of bacteria, viruses, molds, fungus, Lyme, chemical toxins, heavy metal toxins, environmental, pesticides, vaccinations, vitamins and minerals and foods can be evaluated and balanced separately or together. The balance products could be supplements, homeopathic, herbs, essential oils or even foods.

Chapter 15 - The Future of Our Health

Earlier I mentioned the issue of children receiving many vaccinations and being bombarded with the toxins of daily living. What will happen when two adults with these insults marry? What will the resultant offspring be like? What about their offspring and so on down five or ten generations? Will there be genetic issues?

What about the level of toxins in the foods eaten all that time? The water they drink may be more toxic than we can imagine. In this 2017 administration more positive EPA regulations are being eliminated that may affect human and animal lives for generations. When costs and profit have a higher priority than the lives and health of people we are in trouble.

Climate change issues are being questioned by people with no belief in science. "What they feel" is more important than real science. What is the point of having experts and specialists in a field of study if the uneducated, so called leaders, reject the suggestions about the climate changes the world can foresee?

Do they reject the analysis of disease conditions of their doctors? Why are the politicians and climate deniers smarter than the experts? The future of the world and the health of the world population may be based on a stupid, uneducated decision made by one or a handful of opinionated folks.

With climate change what level of viruses, bacteria or molds will be released from the melting of the icy earth as the great melt occurs? Will science be prepared to cope with the new level of toxins that will affect humans and animals in decades?

Epilogue

The concept of quantum energy frequency medicine is fairly new. That does not mean that it should be avoided. EKG and EEG measurements have been done for decades. Allergy pin prick tests on the surface of the skin are done by allergists to see the body reaction to food, plant and animal products. The body reaction to an allergy is seen very quickly. We can "see" the response of the skin scratch test. Acupuncturists use multi-level pulses to determine health issues.

The biofeedback system shows similar responses and reactions to different items, whether it is foods, bacteria, viruses, parasites, organs, chemicals, metals, pesticides, environmental products and even fungus and mold.

The frequency of a product is "tested" by your body and the results are recorded either as OK or as a stress. A list of stressors is created, and we can see body issues based on severity of the stress numbers. Each group of stress items can be tested as a group or each group folder can be opened to specifically see what individual stress item(s) need to be balanced. Opening the groups takes a little longer but it is of interest to the patients. Each individual item in the group can be checked for stress.

The potential of the frequency system is light years ahead of slow laboratory tests which are limited in their scope and range of tests. The biofeedback system can be a tool to be used as the medicine test of the future. It could be the first step before costly and time-consuming tests are scheduled.

When the body says yes to questions asked by the bio-feedback system, we may get a better understanding of what the body needs to stay well, disease free and age gracefully.

Emotions have a major factor in how we feel, how we act and how healthy we are. Emotions can affect our physiology and can affect stress states which can increase inflammation and may even lead to disease conditions. Dr. Gabor Mate, in his book, *"When the Body Says No"*, states "in the latest scientific findings about the role that stress, and individual emotional makeup play in an array of diseases, including heart disease, diabetics, irritable bowel syndrome, multiple sclerosis, arthritis, cancer, ALS, among others."

Richard Earle, PhD states "medical science searches high and low for the causes of cancer, MS, RA, CFS and a host of other conditions one of the most pervasive factors leading to illness is the hidden stresses embedded in our daily lives. Stress can affect our immune defenses."

As you have seen within this text, many stresses in our lives are discussed in the case studies. Stresses are shown by individual patient case studies and then we can see how they are balanced. The biofeedback system is a powerful tool to allow health practitioners to assist patients at a level never seen before. Balancing areas of stress is the first step to allow the body's immune system to work at freeing up immune defenses to attack more important disease states.

As a practitioner of functional medicine and systems analysis of the body, I am looking for that required level of nutrition that can help the body "kick-start" itself and then take steps to heal itself. Is it a vitamin, like B6 (P5P), or biotin, or a mineral, like zinc, magnesium, molybdenum or manganese or selenium, or omega 3 or omega 6 that will start the process going? It can be an essential oil, a homeopathic remedy or a specific group of herbs. It can be digestive enzymes. It can be elimination of a food or a food group.

Let's use the world of nutrition, like vitamins or minerals, available to allow the body to recover. This is the layer needed to build a solid foundation and an initial piece of the puzzle to start addressing the complexity of chronic illness and disease.

Many diseases are made up of more than one component. We need the tools for the body to rebuild itself and we need to address the root cause of the disease state. With the use of the frequency energy tool we can quickly analyze products to balance why you are not feeling well. We may determine the reason for your chronic disease.

If it is a toxin, as stated by Drs. Kuhn and Pizzorno, we can apply some of their strategies and see if that works for you. Remember we are all individuals and need to be treated as such. What is good medicine for you may be not good for me. This includes drugs, foods, homeopathic, vitamins and minerals. "Every patient is different with a unique biochemistry and a set of comorbidities and treatment becomes much more complex than simply assigning an antibiotic or two to whatever supposed infection patients are dealing with." as written by Connie Strasheim "Beyond Antibiotics" p.23 Townsend 7/20/17.

The biofeedback concept has been around, in different forms, for decades. It doesn't state it is a hundred percent perfect solution (what is?). But the success rate is quite high. Is there any tool or system out there that is 100% accurate in the testing and diagnosis? The results of the biofeedback system are far ahead of guessing if a specific product, drug or homeopathic remedy will solve a problem. Dozens of health conditions can be analyzed in minutes and hundreds of remedies can be tested and prioritized in minutes. I believe this is a new revolution in health care and wellness care. William A. Tiller, PhD said that the "future of medicine will be based on controlled energy fields". Dr. John Parks Trowbridge, MD said "just like birth of an island as a volcano spews forth from the depths, birth of a specialty can go unnoticed until it is suddenly there."

Well, I believe the time is now to add the biofeedback system to a medical community that is in need of some changes. Any system that can add to the understanding of the patient's concerns, issues and toxic loads can only help determine what the next steps in treatment should be. The cost of this system and ease of use is not a deterrent.

May the healing frequency be with you!

Harold

Acknowledgements

There are so many people to thank for all I have learned over many years. The doctors and professors in Chiropractic school, the math professors in college, the scientists and mathematicians I worked with at IBM, and the wonderfully bright educators that I was exposed to at the seminars and advanced schooling in nutrition.

Each one has added to my knowledge and development. There are three people I worked with for many years that have left a deep impression on me and my career. As mentors I need to thank Mr. Don Myers, Mr. Bob Price and Mr. Paul Stockelman who had trained me at IBM. Their skills and knowledge were exceptional.

Of course, my thanks go to my wife Susan Steinberg for putting up with my time at the office, the articles I have written and the time writing this book. She helped edit the book and made modifications and suggestions to improve the flow.

Kathy Barr has guided me through the process of publishing the book. Her knowledge made writing the book easier than I had thought.

Dr. Vaughn Cook is the CEO of Zyto and formulated the biofeedback system I am using. The concept of the biofeedback for in-office and remote use is a tool that has many benefits and helps health-conscious people and practitioners.

About the Author

Dr. Harold Steinberg, DC, DACBN, CCN

Biographical Information

Dr. Steinberg earned a Bachelor of Science degree in mathematics, with a minor in chemistry from Brooklyn College, in New York.

He had a 21-year career with IBM as a Systems Engineer and Marketing Representative. After retirement from IBM he attended Life Chiropractic College in Marietta, Georgia and received a Doctor of Chiropractic (D.C.) degree.

While attending Life College he developed an interest in nutrition after taking biochemistry and nutrition classes. After graduation he continued his nutrition education. He received a certificate as a Certified Clinical Nutritionist from IAACN, the International American Associations of Clinical Nutritionists organization and received his Diplomate in Clinical Nutrition (DACBN) from the American Chiropractic Association. His interest in, and study of, nutrition is ongoing.

He has also earned certification as an Advanced Practice Chiropractor in injectable homeopathy and nutrition. The course entailed extensive education in pharmacology and pain management injectable and IV techniques.

He has published papers on nutrition for the New Mexico Chiropractic Association and the Townsend Newsletter, the Examiner of Alternative Medicine, which publishes a print and online magazine about alternative medicine.

Dr. Steinberg taught Anatomy and Physiology at the International institute of Chinese Medicine for 4 years, and at the Santa Fe Community College for 3 years. He has also taught and continues to teach live and dried blood analysis and the use of Zyto biofeedback systems.

His interest in improving the health of his patients lead him to research and continue his education by attending seminars on nutrition, chiropractic, and the latest science in nutritional chemistry.

References

Bland, Jeffrey S., Dr. (2014). The Disease Delusion. New York: Harper-Collins.

Blaylock, Russell, Dr. (1997). Excitotoxins: The Taste that Kills. Santa Fe, NM: Health Press.

Bredesen, Dale E., MD (2017). The End of Alzheimer's. New York: Avery.

D'Adamo, Peter J., Dr. (2016). Eat Right for Your Type. New York: New American Library.

Dufault, Renee Joy, Dr. (2017). Unsafe at any Meal. Garden City Park: Square One Publishers.

Kuhn, Merrily, R.N., N.D., PhD. What is in our Food, CD presentation. Institute for Brain Potential, Los Banos CA.

Mate, Gabor, MD (2003). When the Body Says No. Hoboken, New Jersey: John Wiley & Sons.

Mercola, Joseph, Dr. (2017). Fat for Fuel. Carlsbad, California: Hay House, Inc.

Pizzorno, Joseph, Dr. (2017). The Toxic Solution. New York, N.Y.: Harper One.

Ross, Julia, M.A. (2004). The Mood Cure. New York, N.Y.: Penguin Books.

Wentz, Myron, Dr. (2011). The Healthy Home. New York, N.Y.: Vanguard Press.

Townsend Newsletters.

Scientific American.

Science News.

Discover Magazine

Journal of the Council of Nutrition of the ACA

Index

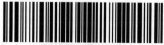

Made in the USA
Lexington, KY
19 April 2018